Trauma Release Formula

The Revolutionary Step-By-Step Program for Eliminating Effects of Childhood Abuse, Trauma, Emotional Pain, and Crippling Inner Stress, to Living in Joy, Without Drugs or Therapy

Anne Margolis
CNM, LM, MSN, BSN, RNC

Second Edition

© Copyright 2020

Table of Contents

Dedication

This book is dedicated to those who are done with suffering and are ready to start healing and create a life they love. It is dedicated to those who want to live fully and vibrantly.

It is dedicated to those who want to take themselves and others higher—no matter what it takes, despite the occasional setbacks—who are willing to play full-out and plow forward despite their fears.

Testimonials

F*or releasing emotions, try Clarity Breathwork. This is a powerful process of healing and transformation [...] that involves generating states of release through hour-long breathing sessions. It deeply supports the clearing away of old energies, patterns, conditioning, and negative thoughts and emotions, and opens the doors wide open for new life and greater consciousness.*

—Kelly Brogan, MD, author of Own Your Self

When Anne first told me about Clarity Breathwork, she showed me how to breathe and said the body can release past traumas, stuck emotions, limiting beliefs, physical pain, anxiety, guilt, resentment, general stress, etc. It helps the body reach an optimum state of being.

A few minutes after I was breathing, my body started shaking. Anne reassured me I was safe and that my body was releasing trauma energy. She softly said, "Keep breathing!" I kept on breathing, and soon I felt something leaving my body that gave me an incredible sense of relief. Then I felt a mix of emotions—I wanted to cry out of happiness, I wanted to laugh, and I felt as if someone (from a higher realm) had touched me, leaving me with a recognition of profound gratitude and peace. I felt blessed to have had such an experience. I was so moved that I immersed myself in Costa Rica to do the full training to become a Clarity Breathwork Practitioner.

—Gladys C.

Many thanks to Anne for helping me out at a very stressful time in my life. I had been dealing with lots of negative self talk, anxiety, worry, fear, and overall stress. After experiencing the rebirthing breathwork, my body let go of a lot of tension and stress that it was holding on to that I was not even aware of. I immediately felt more relaxed, more calm, more at peace.

I think this is a very powerful practice and absolutely loved doing the sessions with Anne. I can see how as daily stressors happen, this breathwork practice is one you could keep up with to basically wipe the slate clean and relax your body and mind. Thank you, Anne, you are amazing!

—Mark K.

Our amazing graduate and practitioner Anne Margolis is sharing the Breath in New York! With her decades-long background as a midwife, she is totally rockin' it with Clarity Breathwork, sending ripples of transformation and healing out far and wide. Thank you, Anne!

—Ashanna Solaris, cofounder of Clarity Breathwork

I've had an incredible experience with Clarity Breathwork. It was as riveting in terms of body sensations as skydiving but with a sense of peace and deep relaxation that has lasted for weeks— and probably will continue for much longer. When I finished the session, I immediately thought, "I want to do it again!" I highly recommend it to anyone!

—Elle

Anne's workshop was incredibly powerful. Something about Anne truly resonated with me. I have attended breathwork events over the years and done some practices sporadically but never before experienced what happened that night. I am interested in learning more and practicing more. During the workshop experience I came away with a clear thought that I needed this as a personal practice and need to offer it.

—Bernadette Pleasant, creator of Femme!,
LiveFemme.com

Dearest Anne, [Your Clarity Breathwork workshop] was AMAZING. Such a powerful night. Thank you, thank you, thank you.

—Ashley Autumn, senior production manager,
The Assemblage

If you ever have a chance to work with Anne Margolis, be sure and take it! Anne has such a gift for holding a compassionate and healing space. After so many years of being a midwife, Anne knows how to support deep opening into vulnerable places and really honors the body's wisdom and timing. She inspires great trust and brings lightness to the work. I felt so safe and unconditionally loved during my session with her, and because of that, I was able to really let go. Thank you, Anne.

—Bridget L.

It has been a pleasure to work with Anne. Her womanly wise and infectious personality made me feel held and safe throughout the whole breathing process, and in her presence I was able to really drop in and go deep. Her countless years of experience as a midwife shine through her presence, intuition, and no-nonsense approach as a breathworker.

—Sophie W.

I had the opportunity to be facilitated in my breathwork sessions with Anne. And I'm so grateful for this opportunity. I loved the energy she brought into the space from the very beginning. I liked the fact that she's a midwife and familiar with homebirth, and a yogini herself, so that brought her in some sensitivity around vulnerable issues and situations within the areas of breathwork.

I felt that she has done a lot of work on herself, which gave her a lot of experience in dealing with different issues that come up. She's very nurturing and caring. I fully trusted her with the most vulnerable secret in my life because she just radiated that trusting feeling and persona.

Authenticity is very important for me because I do believe in the saying, "We can only give what we have." It means for me that if we haven't experienced any pain in our life, we won't be capable to take people into the depth of their pain, and I felt that Anne was always coming from her authenticity, and with that I trusted her. I can fully recommend her to facilitate a Breathwork sessions—private or group—because I know that she will do a great job and that she will be able to take her people into a beautiful deeper journey of healing.

—Ambikha D.

I learned so much about myself, my wife, and my marriage. It's very hard for me to relax because of stress and some health issues, but I got some of the best sleep I've had so far this year! The breathwork was blissful and so relaxing. I felt very emotional and felt some of the heaviness come off my back and neck through the experience. Anne, you are so kind and inspire me with your passion for what you do. What a great group of people we had! I am thankful to have left with a taste of inner joy and new tools to access it regularly. I feel much more hopeful and motivated to sort through my trauma and physical health. Thank you sincerely!

—Jeremy B.

Anne has a warmth and earthiness to her that puts you at ease. She was really supportive and nurturing during my Breathwork sessions and assisted me to go deeper in my process. Anne asked thoughtful questions that led me to greater clarity and to release old programs. She is gentle and made me feel safe and comfortable throughout the sessions. I would recommend her to anyone wanting to heal and release stress or limiting beliefs from their life. Anne is a wonderful breathworker and cares deeply about the people she serves. I would love to do breathwork with her again!

—Asta Kay, Clarity Breathwork Practitioner

Anne's breathwork retreat was something that I never would have imagined. When I experienced my first breathwork session, I felt skeptical and a bit uncomfortable at first. But within about seven minutes of doing the breathwork, I felt a tingling sensation throughout my whole body. I felt emotions that have been repressed for many years. These emotions ranged from fear and sadness to peace and joy. The whole hour of breathing only felt like 15 minutes to me.

Upon awakening, I felt a sense of peace that I don't think I have ever felt before. My mind had no racing thoughts, and for once things were clear. Anne is one of the most incredible people I have ever met. Her positivity, enthusiasm, and energy were qualities I've never experienced in a person. Just being near her energized me and brought about a sense of trust. I absolutely loved the Femme dance as well. I strongly recommend Anne's work to anyone who is struggling to live their lives.

—Valerie R.

Anne, thank you from the bottom of my heart and the depths of my soul for this experience. I was astounded at how much emotional baggage I was able to release over one weekend! Anne is a powerhouse and a firecracker, and I very much enjoyed her style of yoga instruction. She brought so much energy to the Femme! classes that you couldn't help but try to emulate the gusto she encompasses. This was a place to step out of your comfort zone and her presence made that easier. Everything I learned I can use in the comfort of my own home, and I really appreciate these newfound tools for my personal healing journey.

—Nicole M.

The retreat was a great way to begin my path to healing from a painful divorce. Anne and all of the attendees were very welcoming, supportive, and encouraging of each other. Many of the activities were out of my comfort zone, but I didn't feel pressured to do anything I absolutely didn't want to do. The Clarity Breathwork was a very new experience for me, and I was grateful to have Anne's coaching support during the process. After the sessions I did feel I had released some pain and grief, and also gained a sense of peace and joy. The retreat will always be a special part of my life experiences.

—Debbie K.

Acknowledgments

I want to thank my dear beloved friend and colleague Dr. Barbara Gordon-Cohen for being with me through it all, always inspiring me to heal, laugh, play, travel, and do retreats together. She taught me the meaning of true friendship and sisterhood, staying with me through the night of my worst darkness.

I want to thank my husband, Jay, for really being there with me, like a solid, mountainous rock in every storm and every sunshine, devoted, giving, loving, and adoring, supporting me when others doubted, believing in me, and being proud of me—who I became, given what I had been through.

I want to thank my children, such dear, beautiful souls, for everything they do and who they are, and for being my most profound gurus.

I am humbly grateful to G-d for my gifts and my blessings, and also for all the challenges and hardships I endured, as they made me who I am today.

I want to thank Lucy Hamel—who midwifed me through my first rebirthing breathwork session that began the journey of saving my life. I will always remember her wise soul, her kind heart, her provocative, transformative activities she led in our personal and group workshop sessions, her playfulness, and her friendship.

I thank Patsy Brennan, who guided many of my breathwork sessions with devotion and heart, and saw me in my divine magnificence and strength, beyond my self-limiting thoughts and beliefs that simply were not at all true. We became such friends—talking and laughing for hours—beyond the breath. She inspired me to write this book to inspire others.

I am eternally grateful for my teachers and the founders of Clarity Breathwork—Ashanna Solaris and Dana Dharma Devi Delong—living goddesses. Words cannot express my gratitude for all they have done for me and the other souls so blessed to have been touched by them. They are truly healing the world and are a huge source of powerful light—with a rippling effect beyond what any of us could fathom.

I am so thankful to have had the opportunity to take and assist at their incredible workshops and trainings, and I have had many private sessions with them both. When I find gold, I must share it and keep connected to it. They are pure gold. I tell everyone about them and their work. I want to shout out from the rooftops, so all those who need it can access the healing that is their birthright, which is why I do what I do and why I wrote this book.

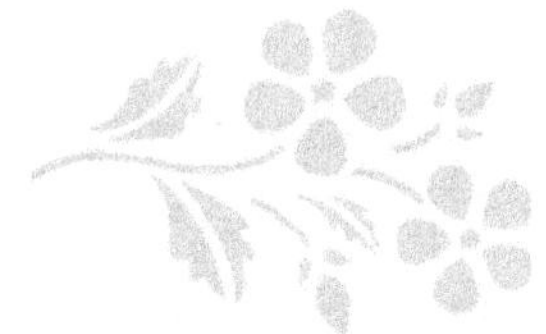

They guided me to release billions of tons of trapped trauma energy in my body, never to return, and to reset my suffering nervous system. I am still amazed by the miracles I experienced. I got myself back—the playful, powerful, ball of joy and love that I am. I found a global community of like-minded sisters and brothers. This healing was so palpable that people noticed, and my relationships and just about every aspect of my life improved immensely. I was so blown away by my recovery that I had to become a practitioner and help others find this relief, deep healing, clarity, forgiveness, and return to themselves and their joy.

I know my healing comes from the profound power of the breathwork, but it was so much more. It was facilitated by their beautiful music and meditations like no other, by the community dancing, the group interactions and activities they led us through, by the safe, sensitive, loving, compassionate, and open environment they created, their sincere passion for this work, and their authenticity. And it was not just me. I was amazed by the healing I witnessed and the similar feelings expressed by the other participants in every group I was blessed to be a part of.

Lastly, I must thank Regena Thomashauer, Mama Gena and her School of Womanly Arts—for her brilliance, her boldness, her outrageousness, and her courage; for believing in me, pushing my edges way past my comfort zone, for empowering me to own my divine feminine gifts and my voice, for helping me to return to myself and my rapturous, sensual joy, love, laughter, fun, and play—so key to healing and living fully; for giving me space to be myself, shine, lead, inspire others, and dance like no one is watching; for pure joy and celebration; and for moving my emotions, all of which I have come to embrace. Her teachings have transformed my life and my relationships and my work. I bring them everywhere.

I want to thank dear Lauren Abrami and the entire devoted staff, the sisterhood they all create, and for the opportunity to be on Team Pleasure, giving back as a volunteer. And Bernadette Pleasant of LiveFemme! They all helped me to recover my life, embrace my emotions, and live fully, sensually, authentically, with vibrant radiance and vitality. I am eternally grateful for that and so much more.

I will forever sing their praises.

Each and every one of you, and the HUGE healing I experienced, are in my gratitude practice every day, and it brings me to tears thinking about it and how I got myself and my life back beyond my wildest dreams, from the pits of hopeless agony.

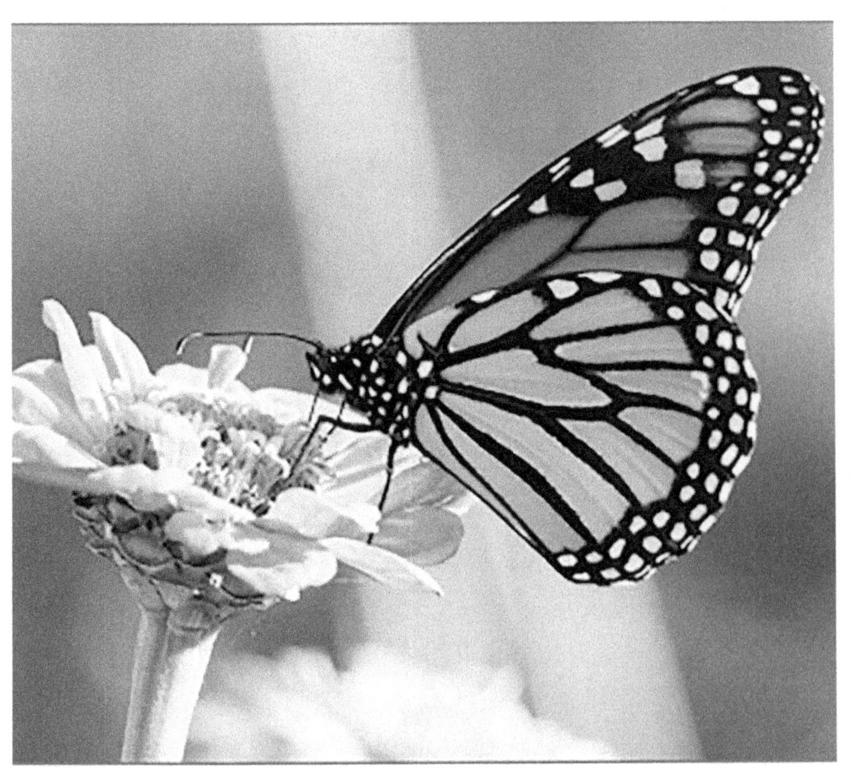

I want to thank my children, such dear, beautiful souls, for everything they do and who they are, and for being my most profound gurus.

Foreword

Anne Margolis has been a dear colleague, close friend, and soulmate since we met more than 25 years ago. We were neighbors and clicked right away, having similar backgrounds and interests. We were busy living our lives unconsciously, going through our routines of working, having children, and raising families. We are both in healing professions—Anne as a holistic midwife/OB/GYN nurse practitioner, yoga teacher and Certified Clarity Breathwork Practitioner, and I as an integrative osteopath physician—and we were taking care of everyone else but ourselves. We awoke gradually and began to journey together into consciousness by traveling to Costa Rica, the Caribbean, and Kripalu Center in Massachusetts for rest and relaxation, yoga, massage, and rebirthing breathwork retreats and workshops, both in search of becoming more peaceful within to face some of our greatest life challenges and to help ourselves, our families, and patients. We needed to take breaks from the intensity of our lives, exploring, living fully, laughing, being ourselves, and healing. Our vacations together became necessities. We took off from our hectic work schedules as we planned, coveted, and guarded that time away with care.

Ahhhh, the taste of freedom, joy, fun, and play. Recharging and restoring. The warm sun and beauty of the tropical Caribbean. We fell apart together and helped each other through our processes. We have been there for each other in tough times and great times, and our healing continues together, no matter where we are. We have been through a lot together, navigating our way as holistic healthcare professionals and mothers.

Anne worked as part of my staff in my integrative medical practice as a nurse practitioner and midwife for many years. We shared a common interest in nutrition, acupuncture, homeopathy, yoga, breathwork, massage, meditation, and osteopathy. We both drew on a variety of alternative modalities to help ourselves and our clients heal, such as Dr. Sarno's method for healing pain, Imago Relationship Therapy, biofeedback, and The Journeywork. Anne advocated for a number of women sexually abused by a member of high clergy, women who sought her guidance despite being threatened. Anne was instrumental in the pursuit of effective justice. I marvel as she helps thousands of women and their families around the world along their journeys to giving birth, teaching yoga for pregnancy and beyond, assisting in the natural process of pregnancy, birth, and postpartum, and guiding Clarity Breathwork sessions with her gentle hands, intuitive wisdom, and beautiful soul.

Anne has endured many of life's enormous challenges, including severe child abuse and abandonment, having a child with a life-threatening illness who survived a bone marrow transplant donated by another one of her children, pressures from practicing midwifery, and living in a family and community that had very different cultural and religious lifestyles from her own but staying committed to keeping her family together, rooted, and stable, to name just a few. Anne has become quite an empowered and inspiring woman who can now use her voice to create a beautiful life for herself and others. She has come into her authentic being and is doing what she really wants to do in life and living every moment with her love, passion, and light shining through. She has learned to navigate the difficulties in her life with positivity, gratitude, and joy.

As you'll find in this book, Anne is involved every step of the way in assisting you to heal emotional wounds and allowing your vessel to be completely free of repressed inner childhood and adult pain, as well guiding you in pregnancy, labor, and postpartum. Her book is transformative and empowering. A must-read!

—Barbara Gordon-Cohen, DO, Integrative Medical Practitioner
**Author of Bridging the Gap to Oneness: Dr. Barbara's
Integrative Guide to Healing and Wholeness
www.DoctorBarbara.com**

A Message from the Cofounder of Clarity Breathwork

In my 25-plus years as a healer and facilitator of others, I have found that the most important key to healing is in the power of our very own breath. Most of us don't breathe fully. We hold our breath and may have been holding it since the first breath if the cord was cut too soon and we were held upside down and spanked. Welcome to the world!

Many of us experienced trauma at our births due to unconscious birthing practices. We were not able to bond fully with our mothers and experience real connection, which is our mammalian birthright. As a result, the vast majority of us experience some degree of loneliness, despair, longing for something we cannot name, and a sense of disconnection, and we suffer from a wide range of depression and anxiety symptoms. Antidepressants and addictions are widespread as a way to escape this pain, and yet they bring their own host of side effects and never seem to get at the root of the real issue and transform it. There is another way!

I've been fortunate enough to lead thousands of people through the profound practice of Clarity Breathwork, which I pioneered and cofounded with Dana DeLong. Together, we have witnessed incredible miracles of healing, integration, and completion of old wounds to support people to open to a greater sense of feeling connected to themselves, others, the world, and the greater mysterious cosmos that we are a part of. We are delighted that Anne Margolis—nurse and midwife—was able to use this work to transform years of abuse and challenges in her life. There is no one better suited than someone who has welcomed thousands of babies into the world and understands the intricacies of birth to help you rebirth yourself as life intended you to be: open, free, and experiencing greater joy and ease in every area of your life. She is a wonderful example that healing is not only possible—it is inevitable when we find the right pathway to support ourselves.

Anne has supported our trainings in Costa Rica and Mt. Shasta, and brings an incredible presence of unconditional love, compassion, and expertise in the unraveling of trauma and opening to more joy! Our amazing graduate and practitioner, Anne Margolis, is sharing the Breath in New York and now globally! With her decades-long background as a midwife, she is totally rockin' it with Clarity Breathwork, sending ripples of transformation and healing out far and wide.

Thank you, Anne!

—Ashanna Solaris
Cofounder of Clarity Breathwork
www.ashannasolaris.com and www.claritybreathwork.com

Introduction to The Trauma Release Formula

Rebirthing yourself after trauma can mean total healing when we learn to embrace the trauma as a transitional life lesson, rather than a life sentence, and when we obtain the keys to healing and transforming our suffering. The idea for this book was birthed from my own trauma and my experiences with others who have endured pain and agony on their road to wellness. I am actually grateful for my own story of trauma and abuse, as it has made me who I am today. As a midwife, I help babies and their parents birth, and as a Certified Clarity Breathwork Practitioner, I help people rebirth themselves, heal their wounds and suffering, and reclaim their inner peace and joy that is all of our birthrights.

For more than 24 years, I have worked as a holistic nurse-midwife, and for many years as a yoga teacher, a Certified Clarity Breathwork practitioner, and then an advanced graduate and volunteer staff member of Mama Gena's School of Womanly Arts. Through my work, I have been blessed to have shared the most intimate experiences with women and their families as they move from being teenagers through adulthood, parenting, and aging.

I have held space for the huge, powerful transformation of birth, that involves challenging situations of extreme intensity, vulnerability, pain of all degrees, the facing of enormous fears head-on, and surrendering to a process far greater than all of us, all of which contributes to the creation of enormous joy, love, and miracles we experience when bringing a baby into the world.

Over many years, the women in my practice, their partners, extended families, and friends have shared with me and sought my guidance for their deepest, darkest sufferings. I would say just about everyone has baggage, past trauma of some sort, emotional pain, and inner stress—that is just part of being human. It comes out as emotional pain, or it may manifest in the form of physical problems.

There is no pain—physical or emotional—that scares me. I am comfortable with it all. I have either felt it myself, witnessed it, or helped others move through and heal from it.

I know that we, as divine human beings, can get through just about anything. You are incredibly resilient—no matter how extreme a trauma you have endured. You are bigger than any fear, resistance, or memory. You are bigger than any pain. You can absolutely normalize and reset entrenched dysfunctional response patterns, no matter how severe the trauma.

If you've experienced intense stress, emotional pain, or any type of trauma, the modality I present in this book is a must for you. It represents sincere hope that saved my life and the lives of countless others. Once you know the key that unlocks the emotional pain and suffering at play in your ongoing personal life, work, and relationships, and the chronic stress-related physical symptoms and illness you likely endure due to it, you will experience such huge relief and powerful healing.

This book is designed to help you release trauma, inner stress, and stuck painful emotional energy through dealing with them in a step-by-step process that allows the gentle tuning of your body to realign with the original state it was in before the trauma and stresses occurred. Stay strong as you work through the lessons in this book and know there is hope on the other side. Using breathwork, emotionally expressive dance, and non-traditional methods of moving the energy of emotional pain, stress, and trauma, along with total self-acceptance—you will see healing almost instantly. Please feel free to contact me to learn more about how you, too, can finally be fully free from the imprints and impacts of intense stress and trauma.

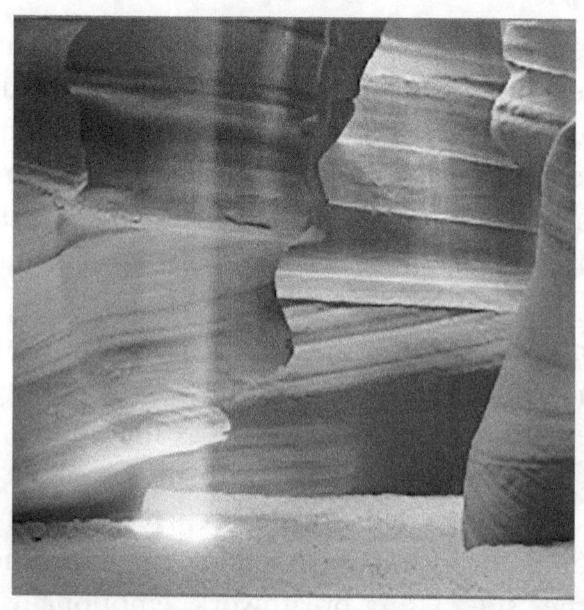

The wound is the place where the light enters you.
—Rumi

As you will soon read, I had a great childhood, a loving, doting family and extended family, and was the only grandchild on both sides. I was a ball of energy, enthusiasm, joy, laughter, fun, and play—and I lit up the room wherever I entered. My world was glorious. Then things changed. In sharing a glimpse of my life story, you can at least get a sense of what it was like to be me, why I am passionate about doing what I do, and see the healing possibilities for you as well; healing modalities that I lay out in this book.

My Personal Trauma Story

Everything Changed

I had a great childhood, a loving family and extended family. My world was glorious. I was an enthusiastic ball of light, joy, play, laughter. And then everything changed. I was nine when my mom lost her mom (my nana) at a young age, quickly, aggressively, and painfully to cancer. My mom became very dark, angry, and scary, and snapped into what I now know to be a serious mental illness called borderline personality disorder (BPD). My mother alternated between a crippling, hopeless despair of a helpless victim whom I needed to rescue and a conniving, terrifying rage of a witch from whom I had to escape. And then, sometimes, I got a glimpse of my loving mother. I walked on eggshells as I never knew who she would be or what she would do.

Around this time, the screaming started, at me and my Dad. And then the abuse. Terrible abuse. My dad and extended family were my haven. But little by little, they moved far away. They had no tools to deal with the horror other than to deny, neglect, escape, and abandon. My dad was a busy doctor, but when he could, he would take me on day-trips and weekend getaways. He played all sorts of games with me. I loved and felt so comforted by my dad, and I cherished those special times we had together.

When he wasn't home, it could be pure terror.

I don't have much memory of my adolescence, but there is one key episode that is vivid in my mind. One day, my dad took me in his arms and said he loved me very much, but was so sorry that he could not live in the house with my mom anymore and had to leave. He planned to live with a new lady he now loved. He was leaving me to go live with her and her three children, four hours away.

"You can always come visit," he said.

My world tumbled down around me. I remember clinging to his ankles, sobbing, begging, and pleading for him not to leave. He picked up his suitcases and walked out of the front door. He was gone. Forever.

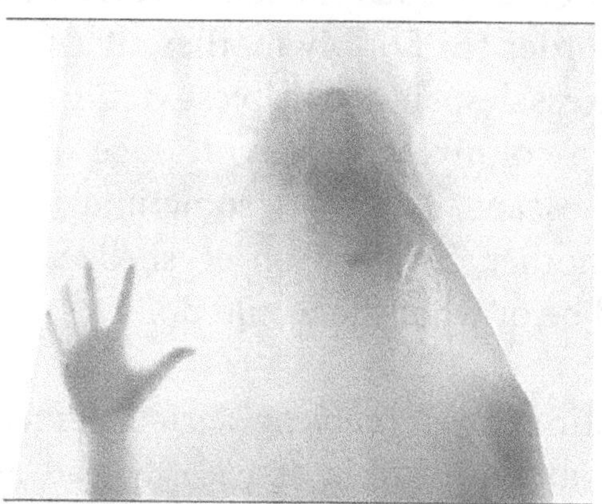

Mom said she loved me. Dad said he loved me. They all said they loved me—but that "love" came with the severe pain of abuse, abandonment, neglect, and the huge loss of my roots, sense of safety, and trust. All of my core needs as a child were blown up and destroyed, leaving me with no solid foundation.

At the time, my baby sister was only eight months old, and I knew I had to protect her too. I had to grow up fast.

My mother committed much of her life to revenge and to ruining my dad. I was not allowed to see him, his family, or even some members of my mother's family that she felt hurt by, as she said they were plotting against us and seeing them would betray her. Of course, I had to see them, so I had to sneak out and lie. All while my insides were on fire. Against my will, I also had to do and say things for my mom for the court case—or else face her terrifying wrath.

I disassociated, buried, repressed, and escaped from it all—what most young teens do—and delved into schoolwork, after-school jobs, team sports, dance, guitar, my friends, and, as I got older, my steady boyfriend. I prayed to G-d (whom I did not know was there) to rescue me.

It was no surprise that I became a young bride. Just out of college, I married a kind, trustworthy, stable, principled man who adored me and had a loving family.

As an adult, I did not remember feeling good or at ease, and I continued to bury myself in busyness to not feel the discomfort and pain inside. I had one huge stress event or trauma after another.

My own "birth trauma story" stands out to me.

My Birth Trauma Story

I was 24 and an obstetric (OB) nurse working in a typical community hospital when I first became pregnant. It was not expected or planned. I was in no way ready to be a mother, but I loved this baby growing in me with all my heart and soul, and I made an unspoken vow from the depths of my being, which was that I would never, ever do to her or any of my future children what my parents had done to me. I never broke my vow.

You'd think I'd have been prepared for labor and delivery, but working in the hospital is where I developed my strong fear of birth in the first place! Let me explain. My family and friends didn't live near me. I didn't know people in my neighborhood where we lived for my husband's work, and I didn't know about doulas or midwives. I felt so alone. I had a lot of fear of birth, and I was really afraid of all the things I witnessed in the hospital as an OB nurse–especially of having major abdominal surgery and that something would go really wrong. I didn't trust birth, the professionals, or myself.

I had no sense that pregnancy and birth were normal and beautiful. As a nurse on the unit, the staff gave me the royal treatment. But it did not feel that way in my body.

I wish I could say that my own birth trauma story is an exception, but unfortunately, it's a common experience still today. I hear it from thousands of women. In most hospitals in the United States, labor is looked at as a catastrophe or disaster waiting to happen, resulting in a potential lawsuit. Childbirth, in the hospital where I worked, felt like an emergency or intensive care situation the majority of the time. It was also like I was working in a factory—get 'em in, get 'em out. I saw a lot of crises. There was no calm, no beauty, no joy, no humanity, no concern for individuals or their feelings. It was about expecting the worst and maintaining protection from litigation. That was my experience.

As an OB nurse, I was actually in more operating rooms than delivery rooms, and I was assisting more cesarean births than I ever thought I would. I was having to rescue women and babies from complications caused by routine medical interventions. It scared me, not just as a nurse but even more as a pregnant mother. This is where birth trauma begins: chronic fear and inner stress are the enemies of childbirth. If a birthing mother is feeling stressed and afraid, she will not labor well, especially if her feelings go unheard and are disregarded. She will need interventions that lead to more problems and a cascade of more interventions.

At the time, I thought this was standard operating procedure. I didn't know what was missing. I just knew it was scary. My hands were tied as a nurse. I didn't trust birth or myself, and because of what I saw as a nurse, I did not trust the doctor or hospital either. My obstetrician was a nice man—my colleague— but the vibes during the short office visits with him were cold, impersonal, and alarming.

Even though I often told my doctor that I felt worried and scared, my feelings were dismissed, as though they were unimportant and irrelevant. I started to think something was wrong with me.

There was no calm, no beauty, no joy, no humanity.

My inside stress only increased from there. When I went into labor, one of the first things I had to do when I got to the hospital was take off my own clothes, and put on a hospital gown. It seemed innocuous then–what we all did. I look back on that now and see the disempowerment and depersonalization. A hospital gown creates a sense of vulnerability, a feeling of being sick, dependent, and becoming an assembly line patient. It just felt wrong: I wasn't a patient, I wasn't sick—I was a birthing mother in labor, but I did not know there were options.

The second thing to happen was I was placed in a bed, lying down, even though I wanted to stand. My body needed to move around, but that was discouraged because the nurse and doctor would be unable to read the monitors placed on me. When a mother is in labor, her body assumes a natural upright, mobile position to help her cope with the intense sensations. And, when you think about this, it only makes sense: in the feat to get your baby to come down and out through your birth canal, gravity is your friend! The pelvic diameter is also smaller when lying flat on your back. The baby is pressing on the cervix to dilate it during labor, and the baby needs to navigate through the pelvis, so your body will want to be up and move around, accommodating your baby's moves in order to facilitate the baby's travel.

I was also attached to an IV and told not to eat food or drink. As any athlete knows without question, if you are about to embark on a long and arduous physical event like running the 26-mile marathon (or labor and giving birth), you do not go without oral fuel and hydration.

My doctor didn't talk to me much or explain things. He just kept giving me frequent internal exams without asking, then telling the results to the nurse outside my room, "She's still four," and finally I heard, "Hang Pit." As a nurse, I knew what that was. I was familiar with the procedures, I knew they were going to give me a medication called Pitocin that would intensify my labor, causing contractions to come more frequently and be much longer and harder than they naturally would.

I was so young and afraid, and I did not feel safe or secure.

When I said no, I did not want Pit, my nurse's well-meaning response was "Honey, you don't want a cesarean, do you?" It was either take the medication or be faced with the possibility of a C-section. So they instilled fear in me rather than knowledge. (I now know that these weren't my only two options, and that my body was capable.) Of course, I did not want a cesarean, so I agreed. I was feared into it.

After that, my coping went out the window. I couldn't deal with the agony brought on by the medication. The doctor came in and walked out again and said, "She's still at a four. Give her an epidural." It seemed like forever, but then they were giving me an epidural anesthetic via a big needle in my back, into the area around my spinal cord.

I was so young and afraid.

All of the things that come naturally are discouraged by most hospitals still today. I was uncomfortable, and I did not feel safe or secure. Not only were my feelings, worries, wants, and needs completely unheard and ignored, but I was also made to stay put when my body was screaming to do what comes naturally ... until it was numb. Then I did not know what was going on in me. I had no sense of control over my own body and my birth. I was in unnecessary pain and discomfort from the Pitocin, which was why I needed an epidural.

My Worst Fear Happened

Suddenly, my worst fear happened. The epidural caused a prolonged and severe drop in my baby's heart rate. There was a frenzied panic around me. I was rushed to an operating room for an emergency cesarean. I was terrified. As a nurse, I knew that if you don't operate within minutes, you could have a damaged or dead baby. I waited, prepped and tied to the operating table in the OR for about an hour, watching the clock, waiting for the assistant surgeon–who never came!

I was left completely alone all that time. My husband wasn't even allowed in the room. I ended up calling out for help because the drugs took over my body, and I needed to push. The doctor came running in, yelling, "Get me a vacuum!" I wound up being cut from the vagina and perineum almost to the anus, and my baby was then vacuumed out. She was pink and vigorous. I was afraid to look at her. I didn't want to see her because I believed that I would be looking at her dead body. They reassured me that she was just fine and told me to look. She was pink, breathing, healthy, and appeared vigorous. She was beautiful.

But I was not fine. I was traumatized.

Postpartum, I had what I now know to be birth trauma, Post-Traumatic Stress Disorder (PTSD)–a normal response to such an intense situation. I had the symptoms, I just did not know what was wrong at the time. I was getting frequent intrusive memories and flashbacks of the experience. Anything that reminded me of the birth triggered horrible feelings in my body. I had a fight-or-flight response whenever I saw a pregnant woman or newborn baby, whenever anyone would ask me about my birth or talk about their birth. I could not discuss any of it without feeling horrible inside. I felt I could not talk about it or be asked about it at all.

I felt wound up, hypervigilant, overprotective, and worried something terrible would happen to her–like the worst could happen any time. I couldn't sleep. Even though I loved her completely and wholly, it was hard to look at her and not be reminded of my birth. Oftentimes I was, and I would cry or feel triggered into a panic. I could not even imagine going back to work and facing the scene. When I had to start thinking about returning to work, I began having nightmares. My adrenaline would pump up, and I would feel sick. I'd be hyper-alert and on-guard all of the time, as I was afraid of the sensations in my body.

We live in a society that tends to repress feelings, so that's what I did.

"You'll get over it," genuinely caring people would say, or they would ask, "What is the big deal? You have a healthy baby." That made me feel worse; like something was really wrong with me, so I felt more ashamed, guilty, alone, and isolated. I stopped telling anyone what I was feeling.

As a new mom experiencing birth trauma that I did not know I had, I sucked it up. We live in a society that tends to repress feelings, so that's what I did. People and medical professionals did not and often still do not take seriously the huge impact of birth on the psychology of women. I repressed and suppressed and tried my best to move on. I am amazed I was able to go back to work, but it was not easy.

I told my husband that I never wanted to have another baby.

It was no surprise, I became pregnant again two years later and started having more panic attacks. With the second birth, I ended up having a very similar experience to my first birth, but this time with a different doctor in the hospital.

Later, when I was telling a friend about my frustrations with the system, she told me I should become a midwife. I literally asked her, "What's a midwife?" There was no internet at that time, so I went to the library to research it. I soaked up the books about it and applied soon after. I was accepted to the oldest nurse-midwifery school in the country.

Midwifery started the journey of healing and coming home to myself.

I was in midwifery school during my third pregnancy. I was still traumatized from my two previous births, but I knew what was possible. I hired an excellent midwife and looked forward to a much better experience the third-time around. I prepared in a whole different way, and I had completely transformed my mindset. My birth team, setting, preparation, and mindset shift were keys to my success.

I told my midwife that for me to authentically practice midwifery, it had to work for me. Honestly, I really did not think I could actually do it: a gentle, joyful natural birth. She reassured me I could, and that it would prove to be healing and empowering.

The experience was as different as night from day in comparison to my previous pregnancies and births. In labor and birth, I wasn't tied down to the bed. It was a relaxed environment. I labored in the tub and in the shower. We played music, and I would dance. She periodically checked my baby's heart rate. The birthing process was beautiful and was treated as something normal rather than a crisis. I wasn't left alone by my midwife. She helped me with her words and her heart, allowing my body to do what it was designed to do. She gave me the trust that my body could do it. I wasn't afraid. I felt very supported.

I wasn't an emergency room patient. I was a strong woman having a baby. It was challenging but so doable. I was encouraged to find my own strength, and I did it! I was so proud of myself. It not only helped to begin to heal my birth trauma, but it also restored my confidence. It also convinced me that midwifery care works and that I could now truly help women as a midwife.

My fourth birth had all these same components and reinforced my awakening, my healing, and passion to help others have these kinds of experiences. I was so relieved after my own last two births in this way. I was filled with elation beyond words.

But as I got older and faced a lot of other big stresses and real traumas, one after another, I just kept repressing and suppressing. It was subconscious. I'd mastered it as a kid. Over and over I got knocked down, but then I got up. I kept it all together.

I had, by now, a very busy midwifery practice and was raising four kids, but I was not feeling well inside. I was midwifing everyone but myself.

The Wakeup Call

The main wakeup call was when my young teenaged daughter was diagnosed with a serious life-threatening illness around the same time her best friend died from something similar.

We tried everything—alternative modalities first, and then conventional treatments. The only treatment to save her life was a bone marrow transplant after high-dosage chemotherapy. One of my young children was the perfect match donor. My daughter miraculously recovered after eight years of hell. And her doctor, chief of bone marrow transplant (BMT) at the hospital, came to her wedding.

But in the midst of it, everything just became too much. I had enough. The mountain was too big. I had nothing left to fight it.

At one point, I fell to the floor writhing in deep emotional pain that just seemed to take over. I wept, and I prayed. I felt no one heard or answered. It was absolute torture to be in my body. I was finally ready to give into it. But—I knew I did not want to stay curled up in a fetal position.

I did not want to be like my poor mother, who has lived her life as a powerless victim, lamenting over all the terrible things that happened to her.

You don't know how strong you are until you have to be that strong. I made a choice to do whatever it took to get myself well, to take myself higher, to be there for myself, my family, my friends, and the families in my practice. There was no other way. I upped my self-care, improved my already-healthy diet, took more dance classes, and tried just about everything—acupuncture, The Journey work, hypnotherapy, massage, biofeedback, supplements, herbs, homeopathy, chiropractic and osteopathic care, and Reiki. I read piles of self-help books and went to numerous healing workshops and retreats. Nothing touched it—not even my more regular and deeper yoga and meditation practices.

I did all sorts of therapy with all sorts of therapists, but talking about it and wallowing in the pain just made it worse.

I eventually went to doctors and psychiatrists who just wanted to drug me. I knew that was not the cure, but I was so desperate I tried a few. The side effects were even more intolerable, and no medication actually helped. Nothing worked. I was not far from giving up, but I couldn't give up. My kids needed me to be well. And it is not in my personality to give up.

I searched for and found a holistic integrative psychiatrist who had a wonderful reputation and came highly recommended. I told her I was going crazy and something was terribly wrong.

She spent almost two hours with me and focused a lot on my childhood, about which I did not have much memory. She said I was not crazy. She nailed it. She said I had chronic PTSD (post traumatic stress disorder), from adult traumas, but more significantly from the years of severe abuse I had experienced as a child through teen years during my most crucial formative development.

I had never used those words before to describe my past, but it made so much sense. She said all the remedies and treatments I had tried did not work because cutting-edge trauma research indicates unprocessed trauma is stored as trapped energy in the body, and it needs to be released from the body with somatic types of therapies—not by talking about it or medication. My central nervous system needed to be reset, as it was in a perpetual state of self-preservation fight or flight, which causes dis-ease and many of the physical and mental health problems of modern living.

Other medical professionals said I was so damaged, I would never heal. She said it was serious, but I absolutely could heal. I was thrilled to get a diagnosis and hope for a cure, and to hear I was not going nuts (even though it felt like it!). She mentioned trauma therapies like Somatic Experience (SE) and Organic Intelligence (OI), Dialectical Behavior Therapy (DBT) and Emotional Freedom Technique (EFT) but first and foremost, I must follow a trauma release and nervous system reset regimen.

Then I needed empowerment, to get back my joy, play, and laughter, and create a life I love—which is an integral part of healing and living fully.

She sent me to her therapist, who led me to another game-changer and life saver—Mama Gena's School of Womanly Arts—where I did all that and more. We made a follow-up appointment, but I felt better already, just knowing this.

The Key to Healing Is Revealed

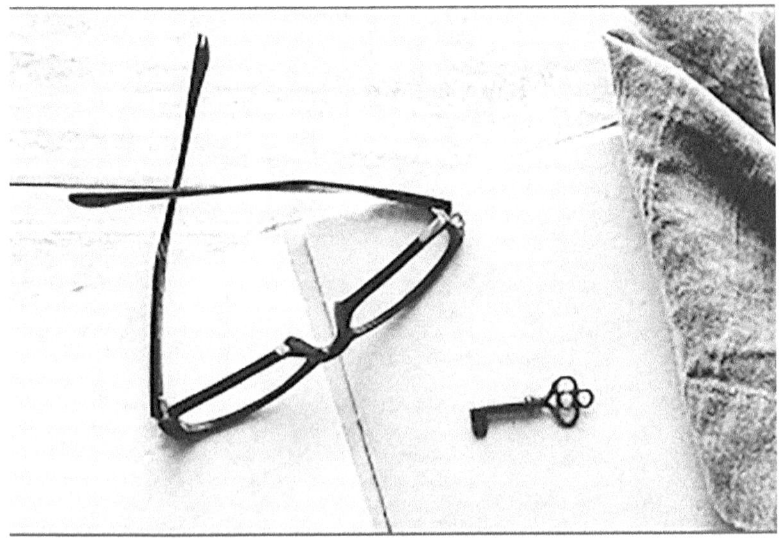

Around that time, I went on a yoga retreat in Costa Rica with a dear friend and colleague. During lunch, a woman on our retreat was sharing how she was blown away and raving about the most powerful healing experience of her life during a breathwork rebirthing session she had with a local practitioner. She said she felt like she released a ton of trauma energy from her body.

I made an appointment right away. And that was the appointment that began the journey that saved my life.

The practitioner, Lucy, spent a lot of time asking me focused questions about my past, as far back as I could remember. She was very wise, kind, and compassionate, but direct and confrontational, which is what I needed. I really did not care at this point. I just wanted to feel better and release whatever was causing my suffering.

My First Breathwork Session

Lucy then led me through a session of continuous, conscious, connective breathing, regular and flowing, but deep, full, and circular. I eventually became semi-conscious—there, but not there. I felt all kinds of interesting sensations. I was scared about them, but she reassured me it was normal healing, to keep focused on the breathing. I felt tingling, electric-like feelings in my feet, legs, arms, and hands that traveled up my body, but stopped at my chest.

It felt like a dark, black, heavy steel wall was there blocking it, making it impossible to penetrate. It felt deep and endless, like a bottomless pit. I did not like this and wanted the things I felt in my heart and chest area to go away. Lucy lovingly said that it was from my years of burying and repressing my intolerable pain. It helped and protected me as a child, but it was not serving me now.

I could release it, if I wanted.

"I can't," I told her.

She said, "Don't try. Just let it be there and breathe."

I was resisting and had trouble letting go.

She midwifed me and guided me, and I surrendered. Eventually, it literally felt like the heavy steel wall dissolved, and then the tingling and electricity traveled all over my body. After that, my whole body started shaking, and I asked her what was happening. She reassured me that it was all good. This was the trauma releasing. "Bring it on!" I remember thinking, and it felt beyond awesome.

When that resolved, my body was as heavy as lead and I could not move, but I did not want to. I also felt the most delicious feeling of relief and lightness within me. Like hundreds of pounds of bricks of trapped trauma energy had just left my body.

I really did not care at that point. I just wanted to feel better and release whatever was causing my suffering.

At the end of the session, it was so powerful. I asked her, "What drug did you just give to me? What did you do to me?"

She answered, "Nothing. That is the power of this kind of breathwork."

I was blown away. I knew I needed more, so she gave me the contact of a breathwork practitioner in my area, and Lucy and I also continued via Skype video sessions. I traveled down to work with her in person a few more times as well.

I even brought my husband, who was enthralled with the miracles he saw in me by doing this modality, and so he started doing it too. I was saving my life—I did not care if I needed to travel, and I was grateful for credit cards.

Patsy, the breathworker I worked within my area, was another blessed beautiful soul, a seasoned rebirthing breathworker who has led private and large group sessions and workshops around the globe for 35 years. I was opening to a whole new world. Each session, I released and healed more and more, and got to deeper places. Healing is like peeling away layers of an onion, and I was committed to giving it my all. It was working. Finally, something was working! I was feeling more and more at ease with my body; more and more myself.

More Release, More Healing

I did not feel done, though, and I was frustrated. I decided to immerse myself in a month-long intensive Clarity Breathwork group program led by Dana Dharma Devi Delong and Ashanna Solaris. It was there that I released just about all of it. Billions and billions of tons of trauma energy left my body, and I knew it was gone forever, never to return.

I healed the traumatized inner child and wounded adult.

I released trauma energy from events that I did not even know were as traumatic as they were, at the time. I got clarity on many parts of my life about what happened to me, about my belief and thought patterns that governed my actions and reactions as well as the results in my life. I learned why I was triggered the way I was, why I made the adult decisions I did. It became clear that I was the only one who could heal myself, and I had the ability and innate power to do so. I had the capacity to rewrite my story, to transform dysfunctional limiting beliefs and lies I had told myself repetitively for so many years. I freed myself from the bondage of false conditioned negative thought patterns.

I had the capacity to rewrite my story.

Without condoning abuse and neglect, I was able to find forgiveness for all those who harmed me, as they either were ill, wounded themselves, or doing the best they could with what they knew and faced at the time. I forgave, loved, and had compassion for myself and for others.

I connected to my own spirituality, to the (loving) divine in me, in each person and all that is. I experienced incredible empowerment, wonderful transformation, and miracles. Every day and every moment I think about it, I am brought to tears of gratitude for this work, for all the living angels who guided me to this place.

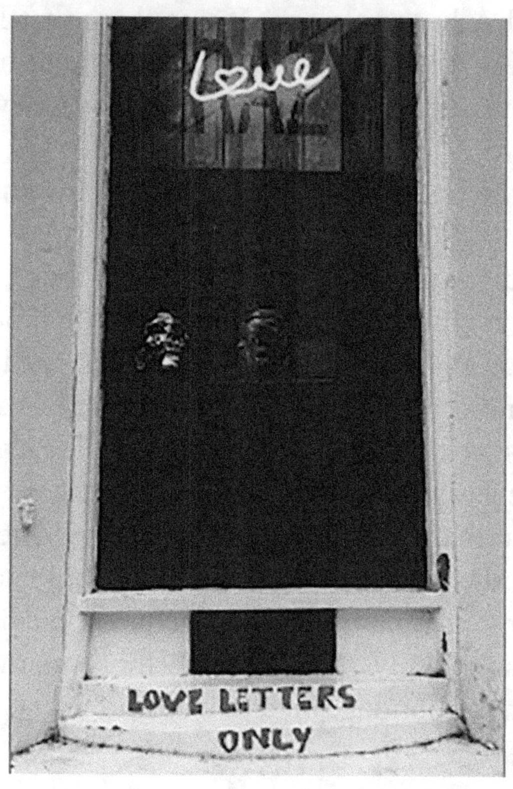

Gold

I found gold and I have to share it! I took the full training and got certified as a Clarity Breathwork practitioner. I studied with world-renowned breathworkers like Dan Brule of Breath Mastery and Judith Kravitz of Transformational Breath. I attended the International Breathwork Conferences, took other training, growth, and transformational workshops to fine-tune my abilities to help others heal their wounds and suffering, and get back their peace and joy.

What is revolutionary is that one key unlocks all locks. I'm going to show you what the key is that unlocks and opens the door to healing your health and wellbeing, your relationships, love life, career, how you feel inside, and the key to ending your suffering, so everything falls into place.

This is what I want for you!

The Trauma Release Formula

The Root Cause

The surface-level issues you are suffering are not the source; the root cause. You have unprocessed energy of traumas, emotional pain, and inner stress on all levels since birth and early childhood onward (possibly even before that—while in the womb), and harmful, repetitive, untrue but very real thought patterns trapped in your body without the technology to release it.

We live in a culture that does not understand or fully acknowledge trauma, what it is and its effect and impact on every aspect of our lives.

Conventional, traditionally-trained medical doctors and psychiatric and psychological therapies and even many common alternative modalities cannot help you.

Your world is a reflection of your internal self.

Subconscious/Unconscious Mind

Most of our thoughts and behaviors are governed by our subconscious/unconscious mind.

The conscious mind that we have access to is only the tip of the vast consciousness iceberg beneath. Everything that has ever happened to us, including our core self-limiting beliefs, repetitive patterns, and conditioning that produce results in our lives, is recorded and contained in our sub/unconscious mind/body—like a highly sophisticated computer. Your world is a reflection of your internal self.

We attract, interpret/project, manifest, and set up situations in our lives in ways that align with our belief system—most of which is subconscious. For example, if we believe we are failures, we will find ways to sabotage our actions and end up failing at what we attempt; if we believe we are not worthy or not enough, we create a life that reinforces that deep-rooted lie. We remain stuck in past traumas without even knowing it. We act out untrue beliefs to prove them true, project them onto everyone and everything, or overcompensate and do anything to prove it wrong, or that it isn't true.

It's Not Your Fault

While it is not your fault how you were born, how you were conditioned and patterned to believe, and what happened to you as a child, and most of what we face in life that is not in our control—it is your responsibility to liberate yourself if you want to heal, be free, and enhance all aspects of your life, including your work and relationships with others.

Maybe therapists, doctors, conventional and alternative modalities were not able to help you, but there are effective revolutionary tools out there, and I'm going to show you how they work so you can apply them in your life.

You will come to understand that those problems that have been getting in the way of your wellbeing and living, keeping you from your most healthy, fulfilled, joyous life and great, loving relationships, keeping you from showing up fully in your personal life and your work often have the same underlying cause(s).

Many of your problems are from trapped energy in your body of unprocessed trauma, emotional pain, inner stress, and repetitive dysfunctional and false thought patterns.

You've read my story and you will soon read the stories of other people, how that happened for them, so you can begin to imagine what the possibility is for you. There is hope!

Why You Have Traumatic Responses

You have **unprocessed energy of traumas**, emotional pain, and inner stress on all levels, and harmful, repetitive, untrue but very real thought patterns trapped in your body without the knowledge to release it. We live in a culture that does not understand or fully acknowledge trauma, what it is, and its effect and impact on every aspect of our lives.

Let's talk more about the stress response and research on the topic.

The Stress Response

Peter A. Levine, PhD, cutting-edge trauma expert, and founder of Somatic Experiencing for trauma healing, points out the following in his best-selling book, In an Unspoken Voice, How the Body Releases Trauma and Restores Goodness:

"Let's go deeper into the stress response, that protects us in acute danger, but can harm us if ongoing without natural resolution.

Traumatic and overwhelming stressful situations of all degrees, where one feels threatened, frightened, and powerless elicits a survival instinct response, in both human beings and animals, so we can escape danger and get to safety. When animals run from a predator, they use the increased energy of the fight or flight response, to flee and protect themselves, and when free of the threat to their lives, they shake and discharge the rest of it off. They involuntarily self-regulate, settle and return to their equilibrium. If the danger is imminent, with little chance of survival, the animal's trauma response is to freeze, shut down, disassociate and anesthetize, as if to play dead, which can ultimately lead to successful escape (the predator often leaves a dead animal they think they acquired, to hunt another) or minimize the pain of attack. Again, if the animal makes it to safety, it shakes and resets and resumes being in the calm, alert optimal state. These are universal instinctual responses of traumatic helplessness in intense overwhelming experiences of extreme danger. What is fascinating is like humans, if the animal's trauma responses are interfered with, there is usually a profound sense of defenselessness associated with increased levels of stress and fear, they can have more difficulty self-regulating. Humans get stuck in a dysfunctional vicious cycle of trauma responses without the original trigger, and without resolution to completion."

Humans Get Stuck in the Trauma Cycle

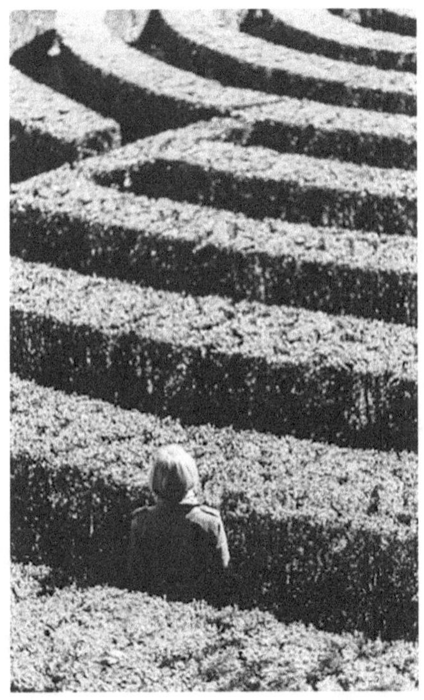

As humans, we often do not allow for our normal intuitive and primal nervous system to go through and complete this full rebound and self-regulating process, and this leaves us more vulnerable to getting stuck in the trauma cycle.

When exposed to reminders and events that trigger it, even when they are not considered traumatic or even upsetting to someone else, we get the fight-or-flight or freeze response when there is nothing to escape from—it becomes our default response to just about any stress. This takes a tremendous toll on our physical and emotional wellbeing over time.

When we are in an increased state of arousal, we do tend to shiver, like if nervous, for example, after giving birth, waking from anesthesia after surgery, upon hearing shocking or terrifying news, after an accident or injury, and even after orgasm, but we are not taught to allow for and embrace it; rather, we are encouraged to stop it, drug it, or talk ourselves out of it. Stopping it is like trying to stop a waterfall. Drugging it then makes no sense, and talking about it does not touch it and does nothing to release the energy or reset the nervous system. When upset, stressed, or even traumatized, we are taught to suppress, escape, numb, and even deny our normal reactions and feelings. This leaves us stuck physically and emotionally, which dominates our lives in many negative ways.

Becoming aware of this normal healthy response to stress and trauma lessens its gripping hold. Allowing and embracing the trauma energy and associated sensations of our reactions to emerge and complete themselves is our path to salvation and freedom from them.

What Are Trauma Symptoms?

The symptoms you experience when the energy of inner stress, pain, and trauma is trapped in your body and your nervous system is stuck in the dysfunctional trauma response are vast, but some are listed here. With each symptom, there are many layers of potential as to what may be inside of the symptom. This revolutionary method of healing trauma will penetrate those layers, so you can heal deeply and fully. Just remember, a high-impact, traumatic, or painful memory is simply that—it is an imprint of something that caused great agony, fear, and helplessness trapped in the cellular memories and subconscious of your body. Everything that has ever happened to us is stored in our vast subconscious that governs our reactions, behavior, and lives—most of which we do have not access to, but the existence of inner stress, pain, and trauma within it is causing all kinds of physical, emotional, personal, and relationship imbalances; it can even cause physical and emotional disease to form, so giving your attention to this healing method will facilitate faster healing in your body and your life.

Symptoms of Trapped Trauma, Emotional Pain, and Inner Stress

1. You often feel stressed out, worried, and anxious. This may seem like a common theme among everyone around you, but when you have endured trauma, these symptoms may be telling you to look inward and inquire about what is causing your suffering.
2. You feel overwhelmed, overworked, depleted, burned out; spending all your time and energy taking care of everyone but yourself. Often, you may even feel like you are walking around in someone's body, and not really connected to your own reality.
3. You are filled with resentment, anger, rage, and other people see and notice this. The feelings of anger and rage were caused by the trauma that is now over, but much of

it was repressed, and it feels as real as if the episode were more recent or keeps happening.

4. You are irritable, cranky, and reactive, even to your loved ones and children. Reactions happen quickly, and you wonder why they occurred. Your nervous system is on overdrive, but this can also be your wounded inner child simply trying to get your attention.

5. You are unhappy, uninspired, unfulfilled, sad, or downright depressed—you do not feel joy and this goes with you everywhere. Even when trying your best to enjoy things you used to love, you feel no pleasure or even feel gloomy. This is an attachment to the imprint of trauma.

6. You are addicted to harmful habits of which you are aware, but cannot seem to stop. Harmful habits range from eating unhealthy foods, sex addiction, overwork, alcohol or drug dependence, to gambling. They often develop to numb the pain inside.

7. You feel embarrassed or ashamed by some part of your body. Seeing yourself in a mirror makes you cringe, and you want to cover it up so others don't notice. This is usually related to false beliefs you developed as a result of the earlier trauma.

8. You may be struggling with eating disorders such as binge eating, guilt eating, or you may not be eating at all. Unhealed emotional pain, inner stress, and trauma are temporarily soothed by a bowl of ice cream, a box of cookies, or a bag of potato chips. You may even decide you just don't want food that you once enjoyed.

9. You experience brain fog and feel stuck and can't make decisions as you could in the past. Thoughts seem severed, leaving you dazed and confused about where they came from or what you were thinking about.

These are just a few of the symptoms you may have with trapped inner stress, emotional pain, and trauma, and there are many more. The trauma lives in a hidden place within your body, mind, heart, and soul being. Without effective treatment, this trauma will take you a lifetime to completely heal, if at all.

I am going to give you some guidance on how you can effectively and permanently release emotional trauma from your body with ease, reset your nervous system, and get yourself back. Yes, you have to feel every sensation that may come up. Be comfortable with the uncomfortable—as there lies your freedom. But you may even find it to be fun. Choose to enjoy your healing process. Let it be easy. Once I felt I was healing, I welcomed and loved every sensation that came up. "Bring it on" was my attitude and the attitude I encourage you to have to get the best healing results.

Now that you have an understanding of trauma—how it manifests in the body, its symptoms, its cyclical nature—let's turn to the Trauma Release Formula so you can get started freeing yourself from that pain.

The Trauma Release Formula

The Trauma Release Formula is based on the concepts I learned when I experienced my miracle journey of trauma healing, attending and assisting at numerous healing and transformational trainings and workshops as a midwife, yoga teacher, and certified Clarity Breathwork Practitioner, and from years of helping countless others in my practice to heal their suffering and get themselves back.

It is a simple six-step process:

1. **Acknowledge the trauma**—recognize the trauma.
2. **Feel the trauma**—the healing is in the feeling.
3. **Release the trauma**—clear your body of trauma energy.
4. **Reset your central nervous system**—allow your body to complete the instinctual trauma response cycle and resume equilibrium.
5. **Cultivate joy, love, and gratitude**—create Your Authentic Joyful Fulfilling Life (YOU).
6. **Address any health issues that can create "mental illness" symptoms**—like medications, drugs, alcohol and other toxic exposures, inflammation, gut and

blood sugar imbalance, gluten and dairy sensitivities, nutritional deficiencies, and thyroid dysfunction.

You will find that this six-step process gives you a map from which to create your own releasing and resetting ritual. The goal is to allow your body to balance itself and heal, reset your nervous system, get the memory of trauma out of your body, and let your body release and clear the trauma energy. Then you get back to yourself so you can cultivate joy and create a life you love. We will address step six at the end, as it is very individual and may not apply to everyone. But once the body is, for all purposes, physiologically healthy, what is truly mind-blowing is that there is one master key that unlocks all locks—that you can reset, release, and heal yourself and your life, to live in your joy by following these simple steps without having to spend thousands upon thousands of dollars on years of endless psychoanalysis, talk therapy, and risky medications. That master key is Clarity Breathwork, the topic of the next section.

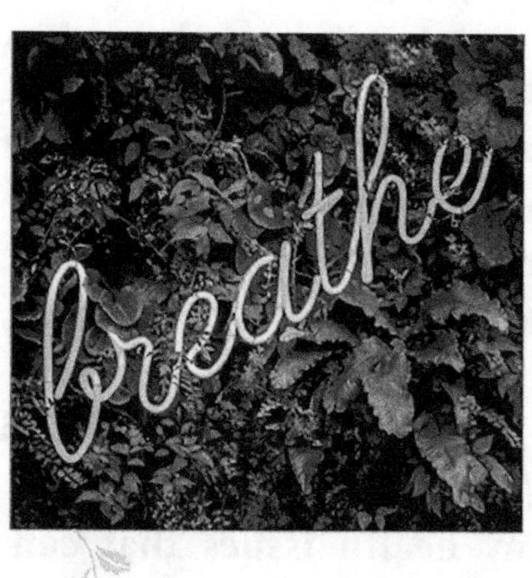

The Master Key: Clarity Breathwork

et's discuss the one key that unlocks all locks. It is breath.

Clarity Breathwork is a potent healing modality, and at the same time gentle and nurturing. It uses a certain type of breath to release from the body the trapped energy of inner stress, trauma, emotional pain, and harmful, repeated thought patterns–resulting in lasting, effective recovery.

The International Breathwork Foundation describes Clarity Breathwork like this:

"[It] is a dynamic body-mind practice using conscious connected breathing techniques for inner peace, enhanced wellbeing, and personal transformation. Breathing, beyond the basic need for survival, acts as a bridge between spirit, mind, and body; between the conscious and the subconscious.

Conscious breathing is one of the quickest ways to open the heart and energize the body. When used in specific ways, breathing allows us to release and resolve emotions, belief systems, stresses, and memories, which are often inaccessible through the more conventional talking therapies."

Clarity Breathwork is a form of what was previously called Rebirthing. It is a safe, easily accessible, and all-natural, but powerfully effective process of self-healing, growth, and transformation that is not usually achieved with traditional therapy and modalities that only involve the logical mind. It enables you to tap into your body's tremendous capacity to rebalance and heal. It increases oxygen and energy flow in the body, and helps gently release toxins, negative thoughts, inner tension and stress, suppressed wounds, painful emotions, and trapped trauma within you. It leads to greater clarity, a deeper sense of knowing, and profound insights into your core life's issues and purpose.

This breathwork, and its life-coaching aspects, can also bring awareness to habitual dysfunctional subconscious beliefs, repetitive patterns, and conditioning, as well as remove blocks and resolve stuck feelings that limit you from living the life you want. It allows for spontaneous completion and resolution of past trauma, emotional pain, inner stress, and stuck chronic issues, and invites you to develop the courage to cultivate acceptance, understanding, reconciliation, and even gratitude for past hurts. It enhances love, compassion, and forgiveness of yourself and others, and inspires you to take responsibility for your life, embrace what is, and let go of trying to control what cannot be controlled.

What is amazing is how Clarity Breathwork can bring awareness to your subconscious—which dictates much of your bodily functions, emotional responses, and behavior.

Clarity Breathwork can even connect you to the spiritual realm within and around you, to reveal the true magnificence of who you are and heal a mistaken sense of separation from these essential components of life. The process creates an incredible feeling of relief, more energy and aliveness, enhanced wellbeing, and real joy. Wonderful inner change creates outer changes in your wellbeing, your life, your direction and sense of purpose, and your relationships.

All healing modalities throughout history, except for modern-day medicine, have respected and included a body, mind, heart, and spirit approach. Let's take a look at how breathwork works on all these levels.

The Physical

Breath is what gives us life, needed fuel, energy, and oxygen. Exhaling is the most effective natural detoxification. Without breath, we die. It automatically sustains our life without us even thinking about it. Clarity Breathwork invites you to breathe consciously, at 100% of your lungs' capacity, accessing 100% of your respiratory system. In modern times, we usually breathe at a far smaller capacity than that, at 20% to 30% of our lung capacity. Oxygen is the main fuel/energy for every cell and organ in your body. During the time you are breathing completely in this way, you are enabling your cells to get fully oxygenated and energized. You are supplying yourself at the maximum.

You are also releasing toxins so that your entire body can work better and operate more efficiently. Your lungs are the main organ of detoxification as well, releasing many toxins, not just carbon dioxide, so you are getting a huge cleansing and natural detoxification with breathwork. Interestingly, it preserves just the right levels of carbon dioxide in the body to dilate your blood vessels and airway passages in your lungs for optimal respiration even on the cellular level. This enables your cells and organs to function at their absolute best.

In the state of breathing in this way, you are bathing in healthy hormones. You are creating a more alkaline state, instead of the acidic state, which is associated with many diseases. You are reducing common chronic inflammation that is responsible for many modern-day ailments and diseases. You stimulate the vagal nerve that activates your parasympathetic nervous system to rest, digest, and heal your body. The diaphragm breathing muscle is attached and intricately connected to many internal organs, so with each full breath, your whole body is breathing and getting the spectacular benefits. Breathwork enables us to change our internal chemistry to improve our physiology!

By engaging in a breathwork practice, everything in your body works better and more efficiently, so you are putting yourself in the most ideal state of health that is possible for you.

The Mental and Emotional

Cutting-edge research confirms what many have known for years–the mind and heart reside in the entire body. Emotions send chemical messages throughout our interconnected systems that link our body to our mind and back again, providing messages critical to human functioning, meaningful survival, and connection. Breathwork is a part of all meditative and martial arts practices, as well as fields of work that require creative mastery and peak performance–and for good reason. The breath is intricately involved in our emotional responses and is literally a bridge between the mind, heart, and body. Every physical state, emotion, and thought has corresponding breathing patterns, which, in turn, impact our physiology. Changing our breath patterns changes our mental and emotional states, and the functioning in our body. Accordingly, we can consciously use breathwork to create our highest, most optimal states possible.

Breath is the vehicle by which we process emotion. Healthy babies (and animals) that are not stressed naturally breathe fully and with adaptive resilience. At rest, their breath is slow and deep, open, flowing, smooth, and gentle without any restriction. When they encounter a momentary upset, they express it completely and then return to baseline.

With societal and cultural conditioning, our natural rhythms are stifled to the point that we can be disconnected from healthy emotional expression. We get many messages not to express emotion, like, "Men don't cry and need to be tough," "Women are too sensitive, emotional, or overreacting," and "We need to keep it together." Additionally, even fully expressing joy is not acceptable.

For older children, teens, and adults, when we are relaxed, we do breathe more slowly and deeply. But when we encounter a stressor, our bodies are still hard-wired to go into the fight-or-flight stress response. Sometimes this can be lifesaving. But if there is no imminent danger, we nevertheless experience all the symptoms and effects of the stress hormones, and it impacts our breathing. During a stressful, upsetting, or traumatic situation, we tend to hold our breath, then breathe more rapidly and shallowly. The unprocessed emotions felt at the time get subconsciously repressed and stored on a somatic level, as trapped energy within the body, without our knowing. This becomes harmful over time with relentless stress, especially if the stress is chronic or severe. Often we are without the tools to fully process it all.

Many people in the modern world operate almost continuously in the fight-or-flight mode even though there is no actual danger from which to flee. Furthermore, they get locked in a chronic stressed-out adrenalized state after years of continuous hyper-arousal. This is made worse by traumatic experiences when a person really did not feel safe, causing tense, restricted breathing patterns and a dysfunctional neuroendocrine system. Operating like this wreaks havoc with their health. Clarity Breathwork is an extremely effective way of releasing stuck emotions and can break the cycle of toxic overdrive, thereby shifting our inner state dramatically. This form of breathwork enables your central nervous system to reset. It is like turning the computer off and on again, so it can return to the ideal original state/intended original factory settings, so your body can rebalance anything out of balance.

Animals, especially mammals, naturally shake off trauma energy after they escape a predator threat and return to their normal relaxed state of being. They move on without being impacted by the trauma experience. The energy of the trauma is not suppressed, so it does not build up and cause disease as it does in humans. Humans tend to carry the baggage of past wounds, hurts, pains, and traumas. Since Clarity Breathwork puts us, as we're breathing, in a semiconscious state, it gets us out of our own way, so that our body naturally releases this baggage of unprocessed past trauma and trapped emotional energy throughout our body and cellular memory; this allows it to come up to be felt, expressed, processed, and cleared/released on its own without having to think, know, mentally understand, analyze, or talk about it, without having to try to make it happen or try to access our subconscious via thought. When it is released, we feel better emotionally as well as physically. Breathwork literally empowers the body to reset, recalibrate, release, rebalance, and heal itself. We are then in a more optimal state of health and wellbeing. It is incredible to feel and to witness the immense relief that follows.

In the process of Clarity Breathwork, you are opening and accessing your subconscious, as well as clearing it of what is not serving you. You get awareness and clarity of your core limiting beliefs, dysfunctional or self-sabotage patterning, and old programming and conditioning, which frees you from them. The power of breathwork enables you to transform them as well.

Divine and Mystical, Breath of Life

Clarity Breathwork even works on a deeper spiritual level, regardless of whether you believe it or not, and is inclusive of all belief systems. Spirituality means a lot of different things to different people. Whatever you believe, it does not matter—G-d, Spirit, Source, energy, Mother Earth, Goddess, Shakti, the Universe. The root of the word "breath," or "inspire," is "in spirit," which can simply be all that which transcends the body.

Around the world in many cultures and religious practices, breath is associated with spirit, G-d, the infinite, and eternal—from all biblical religions where G-d is described as breathing life into the first humans, Adam and Eve, to the yogic traditions describing "prana" (breath) as spiritual life-force energy.

Traditional Chinese medicine calls this undeniable vital life-force energy that infuses our body with life "chi" and for over 3,500 years has worked with it to this day, to unlock the body's potential to cultivate healing, increased vitality, clarity, and inner calm. The ancient yogis in the East for thousands of years, as mentioned, spoke of "prana," breath, as spiritual life force, and have used various types of breathing to create states in the body of deep relaxation, bliss, heat, coolness, vitality, increased energy, and enlightenment–and this is still done around the globe in modern yoga practices.

Clarity Breathwork has no association with any religion or spiritual dogma, but it has spiritual benefits. It enables us to explore, feel deeper into, and connect to the essence of who we are, that which is sublime and so very there but not directly discernible through our five senses. It connects you with the less tangible, transcendent aspects of yourself.

Clarity Breathwork can lead to transcendental and divine mystical experiences. People report they connect with their own higher consciousness, a higher power, and/or the energy/ presence of others who have died or are not nearby, but are still present for reconciliation, support, or guidance. People have reported having healing visions, great clarity, incredible insights, and access to intuitive advice and wisdom.

Breathwork takes you beyond your limiting judgmental mind, beyond your body, beyond the illusion of separation from the divine energy within and around us and each other. It restores the natural mind, body, heart, and spiritual connection. When we remember who we really are, we live from that perspective, our inner and outer worlds are wonderfully transformed, and we see positive change in all areas of our lives.

No wonder leaders in the field of integrative health acknowledge that the future of healing lies in energy medicine. Everything in this world, including you and me, is made up of energy with numerous and varying frequencies. Newton's laws acknowledge that energy changes from one form to another, always moving and changing forms. Emotions are also energy in motion. When this energy becomes stagnant, stuck, or blocked by our interference in its natural expression (resisting, avoiding, escaping, numbing, or suppressing), it gets deeply internalized into our tissues and cells, so that it sends stress signals throughout our body. If suppression of our body's natural energy flow becomes a longstanding pattern, it wreaks havoc within us, leading to serious bodily dysfunction and subsequent physical and psychological disease and illness, which are so prevalent in today's westernized societies. When we allow full feeling and appropriate expression of emotion in our daily lives, through talking, crying/sobbing, laughing, even moving our bodies in exercise, dance, and breathwork, we are freeing stuck, stressful charges and suffocated emotional energy. Returning to our natural state of easy balance is our birthright. When we honor our natural energy patterns, cooperate and work with Source energy, the sky is the limit to what we can achieve.

All forms of breath are contagious. Stressed-out breathing spreads from person or animal just as does slow, deep, relaxed breathing. Breathwork also takes advantage of the universal principle in the scientific laws of physics called "entrainment." This is when two objects or vibrational qualities are in close proximity, they will unite according to the stronger or higher vibrational frequency. If you are literally taking in all this breath, inhaling the spiritual lifeforce fully into your being, especially with the intention to heal, the healing that takes place is all the more profound. It takes in the highest positive vibrational energy and permanently transmutes lower, more negative frequency energy patterns in our body's electromagnetic field. In turn, this leads to phenomenal shifts in our being and lives, shifts that defy understanding. This not only makes this modality even more compelling, but it also provides an incredible tool that you can access at your own will. As the wise holistic physician Ela Manga says:

"[Conscious] breathing is the most powerful, simple, underrated energy management tool that exists … The ability to master the breath offers mastery of energy and of life itself … it ignites the intelligent pulse of life into a blazing energy that flows through every organ, muscle and cell. Life force rides on the back of the breath waking up the mind and body to its full potential."

These unseen but real forces in our world can be harnessed for our own spontaneous healing and transformation. Stating clear intentions–i.e., your deeply positive goals and truest, most lofty desires–and connecting with Spirit at the beginning, during, and before the end of your breathwork session–for example by asking for Divine guidance and support for your session–enables you to co-create with Source or life-force energy and brings spectacular results. All you need to do is open and receive whatever you are meant to. Miracles happen.

Before we look at how to do Clarity Breathwork, we'll first examine 14 other potent breathwork practices. These breathwork practices will help you to build a relationship with the breath to prime you for Clarity Breathwork.

Breathwork Basics– Breathing Consciously

Breathwork begins with increasing awareness about and building a connection and relationship with your breathing, and sometimes it necessitates retraining. Learn to master, work, and play with your breath, so your breathing is all it can be, and you learn how to breathe more fully and effectively without restrictions, to maximize its full restorative and life-enhancing potential.

Start by practicing breathing exercises (options and full descriptions I give later in this chapter) for 10 to 20 minutes, once or twice daily (like before rising in the morning and going to sleep at night), and periodically throughout the day, while waiting, traveling, or whenever you feel triggered, upset, stressed, down, or simply bored. You can do them before eating, performing regular chores and usual activities, as well as when experiencing something beautiful. Practice them regularly so you create new neural pathways, and they become habitual. This way, you can easily use them whenever you face any of life's challenges. Make them your conditioned stress response and use them to change your mental, emotional, and physical states as needed.

These breathwork techniques will give you benefits that are well researched and widely documented. They are simple to do, totally safe, non-toxic, without unhealthy side effects, and health-enhancing, especially if you do them often. They can be done at any time and place, and can help you tremendously in moving through your life with more ease. Breathwork (described below) with extended slow exhales tends to be extremely calming. Other types of Breathwork that you'll soon read more about, like alternate nostril and infinity breathing, are grounding and emotionally balancing. Rapid forced exhaling through the nose, as in the yoga breath of fire, and particularly conscious, connected circular breathing with longer inhales, is more activating and energizing, and can lead to great healing and deeper states of relaxation.

Try each of the first 14 breathing exercises given below for at least three to five minutes by setting a timer. Aim to move through several breath cycles of all the various exercises to really experience each one. Notice how you feel during and after each exercise. Be patient with yourself—you are learning a new skill. Repeat the ones that feel best as often in the day as you can. Choose the breathing technique that helps you the most depending on a given situation. Make these sorts of deep breathing and meditative breath awareness practices a regular part of your daily routine. Remember, you are engaging with these breathwork practices to enhance your health and wellbeing but also to prime yourself for the foundational breathwork practice for healing your trauma: Clarity Breathwork.

To practice the breathing exercises below, sit tall with your buttocks perched upon two folded blankets against the wall or back of a chair; or lie down, supported by a bolster or on a comfortable flat surface without falling asleep (but once you hone these skills, you can do them anywhere). With your eyes softly closed, internally keep your gaze between your eyebrows or towards the tip of your nose; or keep your eyes opened and focused on a nonmoving distant object or place. While breathing, be mindful, observe, and release any muscle tension, working your way slowly from head to toe. Try each technique for a few minutes or through several cycles. Notice how you feel as you relax into these practices. You might like them so much you will continue for longer.

Here are the different conscious breathing practices for you to try out to determine the ones that work particularly well for you. They will help you to be more connected to your breathing and be better prepared for the healing circular breathing of Clarity Breathwork that releases trauma and resets your nervous system.

1. Breath Awareness

Simply watch the details of your breath without changing or attempting to fix them. Notice the inhale, the exhale, the rise and fall of your chest and belly, the coolness of the air going in, the warmth of the air going out, and any other associated details. Explore your sensations as you inhale and exhale, what you are currently seeing, hearing, smelling, feeling, tasting. Just watch without judgment. This brings you to the present and is deliciously relaxing.

2. Ujjayi Breathing

Practice Ujjayi breathing. This is a wonderful natural tranquilizer and awesome for yoga, deep relaxation, and labor. Breathe at the pace and depth that feels right for you by inhaling through your mouth or nose, directing the breath into the back of your throat while slightly constricting it, which makes a sound like ocean waves. It is a calm, slow, and smooth circular version of mild gasping on the inhale and fogging a mirror on the exhale. This is incredibly soothing and meditative when combined with the benefits of breathwork.

3. Triangle Breathing

Inhale for a count of three or four, exhale to the same count of three or four while consciously and deeply relaxing your diaphragm muscle of respiration, as well as all other muscles, then pause for the same count of three or four. As you breathe in this way, picture the inhale as it goes up the side of a triangle, the exhale as it goes down the other side, and the pause as it travels along the bottom of the triangle, completing the shape. This breathing entails getting most aligned with your natural, relaxed breath rhythm, but doing it consciously is powerful.

4. Sigh of Relief Exhaling and Yawning

Breathing expert Dan Brule opines that sighing and yawning are key to mastering breathwork, your state of being and your health. Regularly make or allow yourself to have a full body yawn and stretch several times to give yourself a boost of breath, energy, relaxation, stress relief, detoxification, and improve your overall well-being. It is a natural reflex that animals, babies and children do until they are cultured to stifle it; and science is beginning to discover its benefits. You can trigger it by wiggling your jaw as you take some inhales. Then just let it happen completely. Also make a practice of periodically sighing, making the noise you need without any inhibition. Take a slow, deep inhale through your nose, drawing your breath deep into your belly and stretching the inhalation to your fullest capacity. The exhale happens naturally. But let it be through your mouth with an audible sigh of relief, consciously releasing and relaxing all tension.

5. Deeper, Fuller Breathing

Place one hand on your belly and breathe into that hand, paying more attention to the inhale while letting the exhale happen slowly but naturally. Notice the expansion of your belly into your hand and lower back into its surface, behind, or beneath it. Do this for a minute. Next, place your hands around your lower ribs and breathe into your hands. Notice the ribs expand out to the side into your hands for a minute. After this, place a hand on your chest. Notice the rise of your chest into your hand and the expansion of your upper back into the surface, behind, or beneath you for a minute. With your hands by your sides, draw your breath deep down. Expand your pelvic floor and inflate your entire torso like a balloon with each inhale. Then release even deeper on each exhale as you empty your body of breath. Keep it smooth, fluid, and even. This helps you learn deep abdominal breathing, increasing your lung capacity. To further train yourself in this way, do abdominal three-part breathing.

6. Abdominal Three-Part Breathing

This helps you learn deep abdominal breathing, using the maximum capacity of your lungs. Practice abdominal breathing as much as possible so that it becomes habitual. This is the ideal form of breathing, as opposed to rapid, shallow breathing. Abdominal breathing is a great way to make your breaths deeper, slower, and more regular, so as to calm the nervous system. To learn, place your hands on your belly and concentrate on breathing into them. Imagine a pump expanding your abdomen and lower back, which causes you to inhale. The pump then releases effortlessly, which causes you to exhale. Continue to exhale slowly while consciously releasing all muscle tension, especially in your jaw and diaphragm, i.e., your breathing muscle. Then there is a natural pause until you need to inhale again.

At first, when breathing in and out, keep the ratio of inhalation and exhalation equal. Inhale slowly through your nose for a count of three. Continue to imagine a pump expanding your abdomen and lower back down to your pelvic floor, causing you to inhale. Allow your ribs to expand with air; then inhale air into your upper chest towards your collarbone and shoulders. Exhale slowly through your mouth for a count of three. Release effortlessly, in the same order you inhaled, returning to baseline: your abdomen, ribs, then upper chest. With each exhalation, try to let go and relax even more.

You can play with counts, using a count of four, maybe even increase to five or six. But keep the count of your inhales the same as the count of your exhales by breathing in a one-to-one ratio. For example, as you are trying to master this, count to three as you inhale, then count to three as you exhale. With practice, you can increase the ratio increments to 4:4, 5:5, or 6:6. Then try pausing for one count between each inhale and exhale. Notice that stillness in between inhalation and exhalation.

7. Extended Exhale Breathing

Extend or double the exhale. For example, if you are inhaling to a count of three, then exhale to a count of six, or if you are inhaling to a count of four, then exhale to a count of eight. To take it deeper, imagine the exhale continuing into the pause before the next inhale while you keep releasing, letting go, and relaxing into the stillness. Stay very still while surrendering even more. If you get to the point that you kind of startle or shake a bit, you know you are in the perfect place, that your body is releasing tension and resetting your nervous system. Your body will know when to begin inhaling again.

8. Box Breathing

Another great breathing technique that disengages your conscious attention from thought, relaxes the nervous system, and can be done at any time, is box breathing. With this exercise, you add a timed pause between each inhalation and exhalation.

Inhale deeply into your belly for a count of three. Hold without tension for a count of six. Exhale to a count of six while consciously relaxing more and more. Hold again without tension for a count of three. You can also see how it feels to inhale, hold, exhale and hold to equal counts of four, for example.

9. Varied Ratio Breathing

Play with the ratios and counts of inhalation, exhalation, and the pauses in between them. For example, exhale slowly through your mouth with an audible sigh. Inhale slowly through your nose for a count of four, hold for a count of seven, then exhale through your mouth for a count of eight.

10. Alternate Nostril Breathing

Do this at a pace and depth that is comfortable, with your eyes closed, gazing inward towards the middle of your eyebrows. Place your hand, fingers facing up, by your nose. Occlude your right nostril with your thumb, and inhale through the left nostril. Take your thumb off your right nostril, occlude your left nostril with your pinky finger, then exhale and inhale through your right nostril. Occlude your right nostril with your thumb again as you remove your pinky finger from the left nostril. Exhale, then inhale through your left nostril. Repeat for at least three minutes. You can also then play with combining other Breathwork techniques while doing this, like pausing for a few counts between inhaling and exhaling, while keeping both nostrils occluded until the next exhale, as well as using, for example, the extended exhale breathing. If your nose is stuffed, you can visualize or imagine breathing in this way.

11. Infinity Breathing

As taught in Transformational Breath trainings and workshops, imagine an infinity symbol or a sideways figure eight with the middle point of juncture of the two circles between your eyebrows. Do eight cycles of mouth breathing, with your mind's eye watching a beam of light as it travels from the center, around the infinity symbol, inhaling as the light moves up from the middle and exhaling as the light moves down each side. Then do eight cycles of nose breathing, inhaling as it moves up the outer edges of the circles on each side and exhaling as the light moves down towards the center.

12. Chakra Breathing

There are many ways to breathe up and down through your chakras, but one of my favorites is one that connects you to the higher parts of your being. This is a breath exercise to do once you have cleared most of your lower chakras through the conscious connected breathwork, according to Judith Kravitz, founder of Transformational Breath. While breathing through your nose, imagine a light from your heart center traveling up to the area between your eyebrows, or third eye, then traveling back to the heart in an arc or circle as you exhale. Keep this focus for 10 to 20 breaths. Then do the same sort of breath, but imagine this light traveling from your throat to your crown chakra about about a half-foot above your head as you inhale and back again on the exhale, following an arc or circle. After another 10 to 20 breaths, do this from your third eye to what is called your soul star, one to 1.5 feet above your head with each inhale and back again with each exhale, for 10 to 20 breaths.

13. Forced Exhalation

Another breathing exercise to try is forced exhalation: after a normal breath, try squeezing as much air out as possible, using your intercostal muscles in your chest. Next, allow the breath to come in naturally and deeply, but automatically.

14. Breath of Fire

This is a powerful breathing exercise to practice five to ten minutes daily to destress, detox, energize your body, and harness your power and strength. You will be amazed how it does that when you are practicing yoga or working out. To start, simply inhale deeply and abdominally, then quickly with an equal inhale-to-exhale ratio, pump air out through your nose with your belly by engaging your core–like pushing your navel towards your spine. After a few minutes, take a normal breath.

In the next chapter, we look at how to engage with the fundamental breathwork practice for healing trauma, what I've already identified as the master key: Clarity Breathwork. While the 14 breathwork practices given in this chapter are effective for grounding yourself, energizing yourself, becoming present, and releasing anxiety, it is Clarity Breathwork that harnesses and releases the trauma experience locked in your body's cellular memories. These breathwork practices will help you to build a relationship with the breath, so you'll be primed to fully engage with Clarity Breathwork.

Clarity Breathwork—Conscious, Connected Circular Breathing

Clarity Breathwork is really the core of this book and the master key to your healing. It is transformational or spiritual breathing, the kind of breathing that leads to incredible healing, release of limiting beliefs and habits, and stuck painful emotions or trauma energy. It started in the West with rebirthing and has branched out around the world under a variety of names and styles, like Clarity Breathwork, but the core principles are similar.

It is usually done lying down flat or slightly elevated with a bolster, in a comfortable position, for approximately an hour. You can use pillows, a bolster, and a blanket for support and comfort. I use carefully selected music, verbal supportive guidance, and gentle hands-on support during in-person guided sessions. It can also be done in water—a tub, spring, lake, a calm sea cove—with a practitioner. Water accelerates the process and is an awesome experience. It can be guided online as well, using Skype, Zoom, or FaceTime.

In this practice, the breath is full and deep, but also circular, flowing and continuous, without pause between inhales and exhales. All breathing is done through the mouth wide open and a relaxed jaw. It is literally aiming to engage all of your respiratory system, so that you inhale 100% of air, prana (life-force energy) into your body, enabling the breath to become your medicine.

Clarity Breathwork is simple and accessible to anyone who has lungs. The inhale is enthusiastic and passionate, with full gusto, deep into your chest and belly, sending air towards the back of your throat, to take in a deep, long, and slow full-body breath. The exhale is soft, completely passive, without any force, pushing, control, or effort. As you open your mind, body, heart, and soul, and expand to each breath, you also completely relax and go limp, letting go more and more with each exhale. The inhale is like a gasp, the exhale is like gently fogging a mirror. Together, the inhale and exhale are similar to a silent "ah-ha." To give you a sense of the ratio of inhale to exhale in Clarity Breathwork—it is like 2:1 or 3:1, but don't focus on the numbers. Breathing expert Dan Brule likens each inhale to your absolute maximum and even beyond it, like an archer pulling back on the bow as far as it will go, aiming the arrow at the bullseye, which is your clear intention. That extra stretch naturally triggers the exhale, which simply falls out automatically, and occurs when you let go of the bow or your breath, allowing the arrow of your focus to travel naturally to its destination.

All the while you are staying awake and acutely aware, allowing yourself to go deep and to welcome all sensations and movements that come up as your body processes and releases.

The full and deep continuous breath while totally relaxing into all sensations is really all you need to do. And as you breathe, know that ALL real and honest emotions are positive, sacred, healthy, energizing, and liberating in order to actually allow yourself to feel even the ones we label as negative. Trust the wisdom of your body that never lies. Breathing like this lasts about an hour, and progresses from activation to resolution.

This form of breathwork is designed to activate and unleash the vault on all unprocessed emotions and traumas that have kept your memories safe, secluded, and trapped (which may have served you at the time, but are now obstacles to your wellbeing). This release happens layer by layer, one session at a time, so whatever comes up is simply coming up to be felt, processed, released, transformed, and healed without your needing to be aware of or focused on any attached story. Newcomers need to get comfortable with all emotions, open up, and simply let the emotions be, knowing they will subside. They need to develop trust in the safety of the process, the safety of breathing, feeling, and embracing all the sensations in the body—and that may take some time and practice.

To lessen the intensity in the beginning as you are getting used to the process, you can always slow your breath down and not breathe as deeply, but doing that regularly defeats the purpose–defeats the whole reason why you picked up this book in the first place. The healing comes with leaning into the comings and goings of all feelings without reacting, relaxing into all waves of intense sensations that need to be felt, not resisted or denied expression, before they can resolve on their own.

Once you get deeper into the eye of the storm, there is pure awareness, pure truth consciousness of your eternal essence that you can trust, rather than ego-centric consciousness as distorted as a circus mirror, through which we tend to see and react to our world.

Once you feel safe to breathe fully and feel everything, you can play with augmenting your experience by picking up the pace, inhaling and exhaling through pursed lips like you are sucking in as much as you can through an invisible thick straw. And especially towards the end of your session, periodically take a relaxed breath-hold after an exhale. Relax into the first urge to inhale again, then take a full-body inhalation when you need to, and in a relaxed manner without any tension, hold your breath again. While breath-holding, allow your sensations to intensify and keep your mind acutely focused on your highest intentions for healing and transforming. Let your breath be your medicine and infuse every aspect of your being to give it what it needs—to detox, cleanse, reset, rebalance, rewire your nervous system, transmute all negativity into positivity, and permanently raise your vibration. Feel free to pray for what you desire, but keep it in the affirmative (what you want, not want you don't want).

When all is otherwise healthy and well with you, then throughout the Breathwork, you can practice embracing, relaxing into, and even magnifying intense sensations without the mental story about them. Can you make friends with discomfort and pain in your body and/or in your heart, instead of trying to escape, numb, or fight them? Is there something that these sensations can teach you? Allow yourself to fully feel whatever you feel in your body, including the waves of strong emotions that come and go. Get curious about all of their details, including the borders, edges, and parts of you that feel good or that do not have painful sensations.

Consciously direct breath to any areas of discomfort. As emotional or physical pain intensifies, if you feel overwhelmed or stuck, try harmonic "toning" or loudly voicing chakra syllables, mantras, vowels, or simple affirmative words or sounds, like "Ahhhhh, "Ommmmmm," "Aaaaaay," "Ooooooo", "Eeeeee," "Shhhhhhhh," "Release," "Open," "Trust," or "Let Go." Allow whatever sound feels right to vocalize, making the sound come deep from your belly or diaphragm on an exhale, after a full inhale.

Some find it helpful to imagine black smoke, bricks, or fire to release grief, baggage, and rage, and once clear, then transitioning to a light beam of energy coming from their throat, heart, gut, or the area between the eyebrows, and/or hands and feet when they make these sounds. Know that it will pass, as waves of intense emotion, and even waves of intense physical sensations do during the process of breathwork and emotional/trauma healing.

Experiencing pain is humbling, and it can be a chance for personal growth, instead of succumbing to prevalent societal attitudes that include fear, numbing, medicating, or escaping symptoms of discomfort which ultimately makes things worse. It can be an opportunity to master techniques that will help with the rest of your life.

Techniques like breathing, mindfulness, befriending and relaxing into intense sensations, being with them, surrendering, welcoming, honoring, and listening to them and finding meaning and beneficial purpose in their messages. Pain provides a chance to learn patience, acceptance, and how to prioritize, delegate, and let go of activities of overwork or those that create increased stress, and allow others to help. Yes, there are remedies to help alleviate pain. But you will be amazed how effective this practice is and how much it will help you to better cope with your current pain as well as the pain that is an inevitable part of being human.

Acknowledge the Trauma

In my experience, one of the greatest difficulties for the amazing women and men I have helped over the years to heal past trauma and painful emotional wounds is how they learn to experience dealing with their symptoms as they come up during breathwork sessions—how they face their feelings and fears and feel them head-on. The healing is in the feeling, not the suppressing, denying, escaping, and numbing. What we resist persists, what we allow resolves as a wave that comes to a peak, then subsides. It really works every time, and I am in awe of the power of this work.

Dive head-on into it despite the resistance. It's like birth—at most intense times, women fight it, they think they can't, that something is very wrong, they are afraid of losing control and exploding. Fighting it often holds back the birth and makes it all worse, but when they are encouraged to allow, to go with the waves of sensations, and to let the sensations take over, to surrender, they birth their babies. This is the same with healing emotional pain and trauma. Often, the fear of feeling intense feelings that were never processed is harder to deal with than feeling the actual sensation of the pain and trauma energy itself. The panic you have about feeling the scary feelings of panic, anxiety, and emotional pain will often be your last panic attack, if you allow yourself to feel it all. No matter what type of trauma, from a horrible childbirth experience, to rape, incest, loss, abandonment, physical or verbal abuse, violence, accidents, serious illness, or other acute or chronic intense stress—the trauma will stay trapped inside the body if not released with expert care.

No Risks

There are no risks to breathing fully in this way, and there are no risks to feeling any emotion—all feelings are valid, holy/sacred, and safe to feel and express. Remember, the healing is in the feeling. All you need to do is give yourself permission to play full-out and go for it, dive right in, allow, relax into, and embrace all sensations as normal and healthy and what is needed to process, release, and heal.

There are no risks to tuning into your deepest desires, doing what you really love, what brings you real pleasure and joy as much as possible. For your higher healed self, this would never entail hurting yourself or another.

Clarity Breathwork's effects are felt quickly, and they are permanent. Whatever trauma energy releases during a session does not come back. You get up feeling healthier, mentally, and emotionally clearer and better, more spiritually connected than you already are, and more in tune with that aspect of yourself.

It is recommended you learn this in a series of supported group or private sessions before trying it on your own. Once you master it, do 100 of these breaths daily and periodic hour-long sessions as you need.

Establish Clear Affirmative Intentions

An important practice while breathing in this way is to state and really visualize your desires internally as if they are already happening, by keeping them pure, direct, to the point, and in the present tense. Focus on your highest emotional states as you are breathing, and you can create your desired state. Pick one at a time, and it can change during your session. For example, as you inhale, inside you say or think, "Open," and as you exhale, you say or think, "Relax." Other examples could be:

- I'm safe.
- I've got this.
- Expand.
- Transform.
- I trust. Let go and let G-d.
- I release my past.
- I'm calm.
- I'm perfect or whole.
- I'm fully healed and vibrantly healthy
- My life is perfect.
- I'm blessed.
- I'm Divine.
- I'm free.
- I'm grateful.
- I'm joy.
- I'm love.

Create your own mantra as you breathe and really allow yourself to imagine all the details and sensations of how this new thought feels (what it looks, sounds, smells, tastes, and feels like). Visualize yourself living, in every facet of the phrase or quality you choose, as if it were really happening now. State of mind, high vibrational thoughts, and your spiritual connection can be significant factors in the quality of your breath session and the results you feel from conscious breathing. We need to be very careful about what we say to ourselves repeatedly, as thought is creative and can lead to manifesting our reality. What we say to ourselves—the good stuff and the not so good stuff—we can often make happen. Literally. Never underestimate the power of the spoken word and your inner self-talk. Negativity creates more negativity while positivity creates more positivity. It is that simple.

The most effective visualization is to imagine your dream life, whatever you desire, in all its detail, as if it already happened. Allow yourself to really feel the powerful high energetic vibrational emotions that accompany such an experience. Embody the emotions fully as you did when you were a child. What did you do when you were overflowing with pure joy, freedom, relief, sense of accomplishment, love, gratitude? Do it now, internally.

Forgiveness and Healing the Inner Wounded Child

Forgiveness and healing the inner wounded child are crucial, especially during breathwork. Most of our adult wounds are activations of the earliest of wounds dating back to nonverbal memories from womb time to birth, through newborn to toddlerhood years, and our earliest core relationships with parents, siblings, extended family, caretakers, teachers, and such. Forgiveness never condones heinous acts of harm or hurt inflicted upon us or anyone, but what it does do is free us from the toxic energy of long-held anger and rage, and dysfunctional energy cords between you and others. Essential to this process is recognizing the essential divinity and wholeness of ourselves and others.

When in a deep state of breathwork, and definitely when these feelings come up, imagine looking into the eyes of the highest self of the perpetrator and what you would say to them that you never did. Then imagine what their highest self would say to you, knowing how you feel. Then, what would you say back? Many times when you engage in higher self or soul dialogues, people say they are sorry, express love and forgiveness, knowing that the perpetrator was doing their best with what they knew and faced at the time or that they were seriously troubled, sick, or wounded themselves. Your adult self may need to come into your visualization and give that younger you the tools they did not have then, and your adult self can pick up that younger you at various ages and hold them with love forever in your heart.

Another powerful exercise when in deep breathwork states is to visualize yourself putting on the clothes of a judge, opening the doors to a higher court, and then sitting on the judge's bench. There you see your parents, each member of your family, and every one of these people whom you feel hurt by–including up to the recent past. As you sound your gavel and ask them to rise, each one comes before you to judge them. Look into their higher self's eyes one by one, taking your time, and say as you are continuing the full circular breathing, "I see into your spirit and heart, and that your soul essence is innocent. I forgive and release you completely." Then see the younger you at whatever age they were hurt enter the courtroom and guide them to the judge's seat, so they can sit on your lap in your embrace. Let the younger you also pass judgement on these people one by one, as your adult self did. Then look into your child's eyes and tell them, "I see into your pure spirit and heart, and know you are innocent. I love and forgive you completely and will protect you always." Give them the tools they never had and what they so needed or need at this moment but never received. Some people may need to get in line again to come before you, or you may need to do this a few more times across several sessions.

Once this judgment process feels relatively complete, while immersed in breathwork, imagine you and all earlier stages of yourself at a campfire, with all these past people with whom you still feel a negative energetic charge or tie. Visualize you and them all coming together to hold hands in a circle. Imagine a bubble of light surrounding you. Look at each one, and see them in their own bubble, attached to your bubble by a cord. See your adult self taking out a massive pair of scissors and cutting each cord, one by one, as their bubbles float away into the cosmos.

Ground Yourself After Your Session

Allow breathwork to follow its natural course in your body, of getting the technique, which will take you deeper and deeper within, activating sensations to their peak, embracing them, then release and allowing for integration. Once your session is complete, stay there breathing more slowly and gently, as you slowly come back to the world around you. Open your eyes, feel all points of contact of your body to the surface beneath you, stretch and move your body, even assume the yoga position of child's pose with your forehead on the ground. When you are ready to sit up, imagine a rod of light from your crown going down your spine or roots from your pelvis, extending deep into the earth. Do a few cycles of box, extended exhale, or alternate nostril breathing, and imagine yourself filling and surrounded by a healing light or divine loving energy. And give yourself a soul-nurturing hug.

Stories of Healing: Up Next

Up next in the book are some examples of how Clarity Breathwork has helped others in my practice. You are not alone. Many people suffer, but the good news is that you are here, and you have found the ultimate key! First, you acknowledge the trauma, then work to release it, reset your central nervous system to go on to heal, sense the magnificent self you really are and experience joy again.

Three Stories of Healing

While I have helped countless people on their healing journey, here are the healing stories of three individuals. I share these, so you can see what is possible for you.

Finding Joy and Freedom from Pain

I worked with a dad who had previously hired me to help him and his wife birth two of their babies. He was having marriage problems. He was unhappy, struggling, and unable to express his feelings or feel intimacy. He was not enjoying intimacy, and he was way too overprotective with his children. When he was a child, he had a nanny who sexually abused him for years. He never told anyone, not even his wife or parents. The nanny had threatened him and told him that his parents would never believe him. He really didn't think anyone would believe him, and he repressed his feelings. At age 40, he was tired of suffering and ready to do the work.

He was in physical pain as well. He had chronic inflammation in major joints, and none of the multiple medical and holistic providers he had consulted were able to help him. It impaired his ability to work, exercise, and seriously impacted his personal life. After a series of Clarity Breathwork sessions, he released the trauma and emotional pain trapped in his body, and all of the joint pain went away. Our mind and body are intricately connected. Clarity Breathwork healed something that no other practitioner or modality could heal!

He forgave his parents and told his mother, who did believe and support him. While his father was deceased, he was able to visualize a reconciliation with his dad for closure. While not condoning the abuse, he let the toxic energy of the nanny go; he acknowledged that she was either severely ill, disturbed, abused, or wounded herself.

After Clarity Breathwork, he felt more at ease, relieved, and got his joy back, which improved his marriage and deepened their relationship. He even became more connected to his children and loosened up his overprotective grip on them. He became renewed, lighter, more playful, and loving. He was grateful to be alive and for all the blessings in his life.

A Return to Trust and Joy

I helped a woman who suffered from depression, anxiety, insomnia, acid reflux, and migraines. Nothing was working for her. She felt stuck in a bad marriage and was afraid to leave because of her children. When she was a child, she had a little sister who was born with Down syndrome. She loved her little sister, but at age four, she was told the baby had died. Thirty years later, she found out her parents had lied to her and that her sister was alive and had been placed in an institution. Not only did she suffer from the loss of her little sister, but

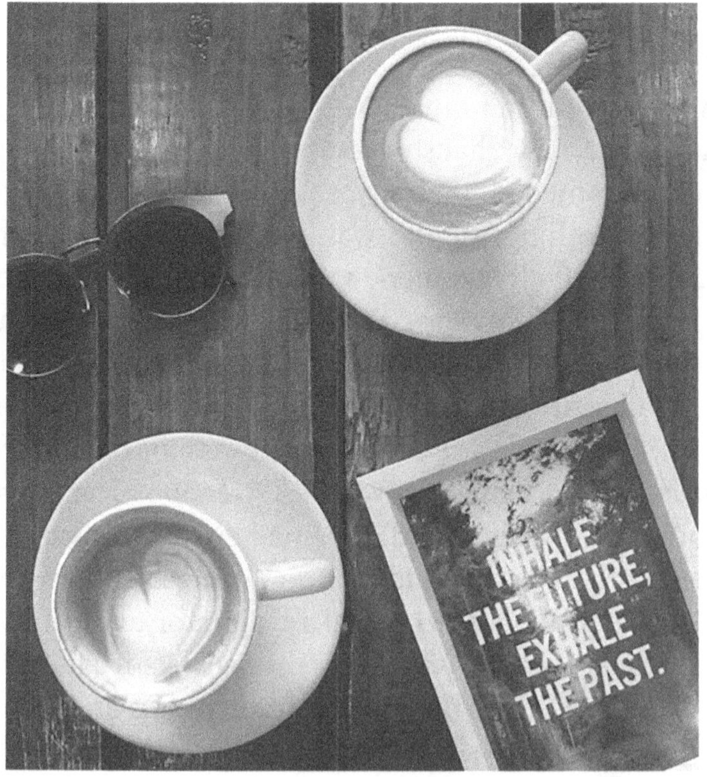

her family also buried their own depression and inability to cope with her sister's condition and had lied to her, and she felt betrayed.

During a series of Clarity Breathwork sessions, she released the trauma energy and deep pain of it all, forgave her parents, and no longer felt depressed or anxious. She started doing what she loved, felt better, and slept better without any migraines.

She is now visiting her sister weekly and is very close to her. Her marriage is on the mend, and she is focused on it with more clarity, love, compassion, transparency, and is more tuned into her family.

Healing Birth Trauma

I worked with a woman who was a self-admitted work-alcoholic. She was exhausted, overweight, worried, stressed to the max, ashamed of her body, and found herself eating more and more. Nothing she did was ever good enough. She was trying to keep it all together—working two full-time jobs and taking care of her only son, who had a condition on the autistic spectrum, which started a day after a routine vaccine. She felt she had failed at natural childbirth when a nurse told her that she was not trying hard enough and was not coping well, so she gave up and ended up with a C-section. The anesthetic did not work, so she felt and screamed during the agony of the surgery until it was too much to bear—and then they gave her so much medication, she needed a respirator to breathe. With all the medications she was given, she was too drugged to hold her baby right after birth. She was traumatized and terrorized by her experience, so she never had another child. She blamed and loathed herself because she really wanted to have more children.

During Clarity Breathwork, she released the birth trauma energy, envisioned giving birth naturally, and saw herself holding her newborn baby as soon as he was born. She imagined healing her cesarean scar and breathed out the trauma, pain, grief, and anger of raising a son with autism. She reconnected with her spirituality and is loving herself with compassion. She is allowing herself to feel more, embrace her emotions, let go of one of her jobs, and now finds time to relax and even play. Her marriage has improved, and she is eating more healthfully and returned to her normal weight.

Trauma manifests in many ways. It may be expressed by emotional pain, inner stress, physical problems, illness, or relationship and life issues. Trauma can exist in the body, even if there doesn't appear to be any history of physical, sexual, or verbal abuse.

Suppressed Trauma Symptoms

To summarize some of the symptoms caused by trapped trauma and emotional pain, many people say they are:

- Stressed out, worried, anxious
- Overwhelmed, overworked, depleted, burned out, taking care of everyone but themselves
- Filled with resentment, anger, rage
- Irritable, cranky, reactive
- Unhappy, uninspired, unfulfilled, sad, downright depressed, or unable to feel joy
- Addicted to harmful habits and not taking much care of themselves
- Suffering from body shame and embarrassment
- Struggling with eating disorders
- Stuck, unable to make decisions
- Disconnected from self and others
- Shut down, feeling powerless, without a voice
- Having a vague longing for something more and better, unsure what they really want or thinking something outside themselves will rescue them and make them happy
- Feeling self-loathing, self-doubt, unworthy, not valued, or good enough, like a failure

- Filled with shame, blame, or a sense of being wrong
- Lonely and isolated–without community, even within their family or circle of friends
- Sensually and sexually shut down and turned off
- Having relationship issues and troubles
- Struggling with career and work problems
- Suffering ongoing symptoms or chronic health conditions from body aches and pains, to migraines, intestinal issues, acid reflux, trouble sleeping, high blood pressure, heart disease, autoimmune disorders, cancer … the list goes on.

If you can relate or have some of these feelings or issues, you are in the right place.

Clarity Breathwork Is for You:

- If you have any of these feelings or issues, as I and my clients did.
- If you have physical or emotional symptoms that modern medicine or other modalities can't diagnose or heal.
- If you experienced trauma of any kind, emotional pain, or inner stress that impacts your life today.
- If you feel stuck, feel like you have emotional blocks, or engage in negative self-talk, beliefs, or habitual behaviors that limit you.
- If you want healthy, natural ways to reduce internal stress, heal from emotional pain and trauma in a way that lasts.
- If you want increased energy, vitality, to feel like yourself again.
- If you want more ease, flow, and joy in your life and relationships.

- If you have physical and/or emotional problems that have not responded to the treatments and therapies you tried.

The reasons you have not been able to heal, and feel stuck in making progress in your life are often because these main causes have not been addressed at all.

Start Your Own Healing Plan in Adjunct, To Support Your Breathwork

Dance Those Traumatic Memories OUT!

In this section of the book, I give other practices that work powerfully with Clarity Breathwork to assist you in your healing journey. These practices include dance, affirmations, identifying limiting self-beliefs, free-flow writing, and journaling. We begin by looking at dance.

For those of you who do not know me—I love to dance.

Dance has always been a powerful tool in my life. I dance when I need to recharge and recalibrate when times get tough or just to get out of my head and into my body–where I feel so much better and more vibrant and alive. I dance when I need to feel and express emotion, relieve stress, or simply create fun and yummy happy feelings.

Because I want to invite you to tap into your joy, your play, your aliveness, even your sensuality and sassiness—all an integral part of healing and living fully, I want to encourage you to dance. Dancing is a shortcut to creating your happy. It's contagious.

It is a great way to relieve stress, and it can easily transform the energy of feeling stuck, in a funk, or bad mood—into playful joyfulness.

Daily Practice

It's my daily practice—I do it everywhere: at home with my kids, cooking and cleaning, at work with clients and colleagues, offices, stores and markets, busy city street corners and crosswalks, with people in labor at all hours, home or hospital. I have assisted many moms to dance their babies out. I've been to multiple trauma and healing, growth and transformation workshops and trainings with ten, 40, 100, 500, and even 2,500 people feeling, expressing, moving through, and dancing the full range of human emotions—grief, anger, exuberance, sensuality, joy, wild fun, and play.

Indigenous cultures around the world and throughout history use(d) music, vocalization, and movement to feel, express, and move emotion in the community–celebration and ecstasy, as well as grief and rage.

Let It Out

Babies and toddlers do not doubt their magnificence. They are total love, comfortable and proud being themselves. They know they are awesome, beautiful, lovable, worthy, and valued. They exude love and trust life–unless it is not trustworthy. And they express how they feel with their whole body.

As babies and toddlers, little boys and girls, we authentically, innocently, and proudly had raging temper tantrums to feel, express, and move through sadness and anger. We screamed, sobbed, writhed around, stomped, banged, pounded, and kicked. We released, reset, then got up and went back to playing. When we were excited and joyous, we skipped, danced, sang, and shouted with glee just the same. When full of stress, we played harder, got rowdy, climbed the walls, and moved the energy.

When were we told to shut down, tune out, turn off, disembody, and disconnect from ourselves and keep it in? When were we told that feeling sadness or anger is wrong? When were we told not to express how we feel? When were we told expressing elation is bad too? When did we stop loving ourselves and others like we did as babies?

There is hope. WE CAN absolutely TRANSFORM THIS as adults.

SO–I invite you to get more into your body, out of your mind, and let the words and beat move you, however it does, wherever it takes you.

Go deep. Explore how you feel and express. You are your emotions with music and dance. Vocalize if needed—get into it, let it all go, and dance like no one is watching. Start in a private room in your home, just dim the lights and blast the music. Soon, you will feel more and more at ease with it. Then once you are comfortable, try it at work or just about anywhere, really.

Channel your little girl or boy, which means be comfortable in your body. Innocently, authentically, proudly, and even sensually, express and be yourself. If it feels silly and awkward, then you're going in the right direction. Even though there is no wrong, right, mirrors, performance, video–fire the inner critic. This authentic way of being is something to cultivate if you are not used to it, but your body already knows. If you need guidance, you can watch others dancing with passion on dance videos or in my group events for the moment, but I really want to encourage you to explore you.

SO let's get down! Push your edges—growth is always just beyond the comfort zone.

Move, Dance, Feel

Dance your emotions, feel and move them through your body. Feeling, expressing, and moving the energy of emotions through your body is a big component of healing and then creating happy energy and life.

Make a playlist of songs in four categories, those that are sad, angry, loving, then happy and upbeat. If in doubt, use a playlist of African drumming–it has a way of inviting more deep primal movement and release. Commit to a time that works for you each day. Play these four types of songs: one or two songs of each type. Get into the music, get out of your thinking mind, and go deep within, explore the way your body naturally feels, moves, and expresses the full range of emotions through music and dance. No prior dance experience is necessary!

Play a really sad song—feel the song, the words, the grief. Sob, roll around the floor, and let the music reach your soul and move your body spontaneously and even sensually through the sadness.

Play a really angry song—feel the song, the words, and have a full-blown temper tantrum. Stomp or writhe around the floor, roar/scream/curse, push/press against a wall, stagger, crawl, kick and punch a cushion/pillow/sofa/yoga bolster, and bang a pillow or belt against the floor or sofa.

Play a love song—imagine singing it to yourself, caressing every part of your precious body. Hug yourself and sing it to yourself as if you were singing it to someone you love with all your heart and soul—like your child, your inner child, or you at any age, even now. If you want to, play with your inner sensual self, move nice and slow, mindfully—you can massage yourself naked with scented almond or coconut oil.

Play an upbeat happy song—shake, move, do hip and head circles. There are so many choices for songs here. Pick what makes YOU feel good, vibrant, fully alive, sexy, and sensual.

Always end with the love song and upbeat song, so you don't get stuck in the muck. But let the dancing tell your story, expressing your feelings and the joy you want to create.

For powerful group experiences, look for Femme!, African drum circles, or other similar types of movement like Ecstatic Dance or Journey Dance in your area. Set to live African drumming, these experiences are an opportunity to find an outlet for deep emotional healing.

They create a sacred, safe space for every participant to feel and live fully as human beings; to move in sensual ways, to explore and release emotions, to change beliefs about themselves and to unapologetically love their bodies. They invite everyone to reclaim their power and to boldly display that power as they move freely and fabulously throughout the world and to radiate our unique magnificence through our body, in every aspect of our lives. The hypnotic pulse of drumming moves dancers and drummers into a joyful celebration of life and provides a space for self-expression of the full range of emotion and incredible release. The focus is on "heart and soul drumming" as an avenue for individual spiritual deepening, healing, and collective community building. It is a timeless tradition common to so many different cultures. An opportunity to unite a community as each individual enjoys a stronger connection with spirit.

Affirmations, Self-Talk, and Changing Limiting Beliefs

Among the most powerful methods to complement healing trauma and emotional pain, in addition to Breathwork and body movement—is regular practices to engage in positive self-talk, and to transform your limiting beliefs.

Scientific research tells us we have 50,000 to 70,000 thoughts per day, and most are unconscious—imprints, patterns, old programming, and non-verbal and childhood memories from birth, early childhood, family, and cultural conditioning. If a thought supports, empowers, inspires, and leads to good or uplifting feelings, then let it flow. If your internal dialogue leads you to feel more stressed, anxious, unhappy, upset, not good enough, victimized, or limited, and increases suffering in any way, drop it like a hot potato.

Know you can avoid going down a slippery slope and that you have the power to turn off the spiraling record player of negativity.

It takes great personal work to replace those lower vibration thoughts with higher ones that are actually more true and supportive, but Breathwork will transform them and regular practice with affirmations will enhance your daily life immensely. You can more quickly turn those negative, often false thoughts around to the opposite when combining daily affirmations with breathwork.

For every self-limiting thought you notice that proceeds emotional pain—write it down and consider how it is not true at all. Write the opposite of that thought and feel that to be more true. For example, if you think, "I am not good enough," note the complete opposite, write, and imagine what it FEELS like to say, "I am good enough, I am perfectly imperfect just as I am and I am doing the best I can," and sit with that.

If you think, "I'm damaged from trauma and will never heal," simply turn that around to "I'm not damaged and can fully heal." Ponder how it feels to tell yourself lies that make you suffer or truths that empower or make you feel well.

If your inner record player keeps playing, "I'm weak and have no more strength to handle this," see how it feels to change the song to "I'm strong." If it is playing, "That ruined my life," try on, "That was just what I needed" (usually for my growth or evolution as a human being). If it is playing, "They should not have done that or that should not have happened," change it to, "They should have done that or that should have happened" because it did happen, they did do it, so it was actually meant to happen (without condoning harmful actions that were done by someone). It is a high spiritual level to realize the perfection in all that is and literally love what is, knowing Source or Spirit or G-d is pure love and beneficence and that we are spiritual beings on a human journey of growth and enlightenment, without knowing or understanding much of the full picture.

Changing Limiting Beliefs

Here are some common limiting, false beliefs you can work with to practice changing them. Remember to change the negative language to positive, empowering language that more aligns with truth, especially during the Breathwork. Here are those common limiting, false beliefs:

- I'm not safe, it's not safe to be here or in my body.
- I can't trust anyone. I'm separate and alone, or different and never fit in.
- No one loves or cares about me.
- Pleasure or love leads to pain.
- Life is hard, a battle, or a struggle.
- I can't make it without pain or difficulty.
- I'm wrong, not good enough, or they're wrong or not good enough.
- It's all my fault, or it's all their fault.
- I hurt people, or people hurt me.
- No one loves me, I am not loved or wanted.
- I'm too this or that.
- Something is wrong with me, I am broken or damaged.
- I will never heal.
- I don't want to be here in this life.

Once we release the trapped trauma and thought energy causing our dis-ease and suffering, part of this work is realizing most of the thoughts we think over and over again, that those things we came to believe about ourselves are not really our own, and they are not true at all.

What we concentrate on expands–energy flows where the mind goes (negative low vibration thought limits us and creates negative results; positive higher vibration thought creates expansive, enhancing results in our lives). When we become aware of this, they have less and less power over us, and we have the ability to decide what thoughts we want to believe, how we can change them, and we can decide to think the new, positive thoughts repetitively instead of the habitual self-sabotaging thoughts.

That's when there is magnificent transformation. To learn more about rewiring your brain and reconditioning yourself to make lasting transformational change in this arena, visit drjoedispenza.com. Dr. Joe Dispenza, teaches thousands around the world with unparalleled success, using the latest scientific research, how to heal a variety of serious chronic diseases and lead more fulfilled lives by the power of creative thought alone. Visualization takes advantage of the fact that a vivid mental imagined experience has a similar effect in the body as an actual one.

It is powerful enough to change mental and emotional states, neurological circuitry, genetic expression, hormone production, turn off and on receptor sites and make proteins that are responsible for all bodily functions. The body literally experiences what the mind believes.

As in meditation and breathwork, it takes practice, with results dependent on the more you practice and hone your abilities.

When we let out the trauma/negative thought energy and transmute our stories of limitations, there is huge relief, freedom, and space. Part of this work is tuning in to our inner wisdom, what we really feel, love, deeply desire, and are passionate and enthusiastic about, and then living from that place. We find our truth, our gifts, our purpose, and we can more effectively manifest what we want to attract and create in our life—and then do our part to make it happen.

When we are aligned with who we really are, lit up, turned on, and excited about living and doing what we truly love and came here to do, we bring ourselves and others higher; when we are not, we bring ourselves and others down.

Free-Flow Writing and Journaling

I highly recommend free-flow writing and journaling, or making art of your feelings. Create a running super-journal of your journey. The Journey Journal will help you document emotional triggers, create forgiveness, get clarity, and heal the experience. And it helps you track your experiences while breathing and your progress.

Here are some helpful guided practices as well.

How to Cultivate Daily Joy with Your Journal

You can create a daily cultivation of joy. Write ten things you love about yourself, ten things you are or did that you are proud of, ten things for which you are grateful, ten things you deeply desire, that you would love being, doing, or having—each with one or two steps in the direction of manifesting and making it happen. Track your results. Note your shifts, how you are feeling, progress over time—one week, one month, three months, six months, one year. You will be amazed by the results of this inner work.

It is one of the most effective, yet simple things you can do to help lift your mind, body, and soul. Positivity creates more positivity. Joy creates more joy. It is that simple.

Turn to the back of the book and begin your journal. Write, draw, make a collage ... whatever moves you!

Letter Writing

Some benefit after inner child healing while doing the conscious connected breathing from communicating in writing, first to get out the charge, then to comfort your younger self and cultivate their forgiveness. Write an angry letter to someone who you feel has hurt you. Let it out—everything you would say if you had your voice; what you could not say at the time. Burn or shred it. Write a second letter to that younger you, a letter of loving comfort and compassionate support, giving them coping tools and wisdom that you did not have then.

Write a third letter back to you, imagining from that person what in their higher fully evolved self would say to you if they knew what you felt. Write a forgiveness letter back to that person, from your higher self, without condoning harmful behavior—to free yourself from the poison. You are free to keep this private ... but consider sharing it with the perpetrator and how that would help you heal.

Start Your Own Daily Healing Process Now

Start Your Own Daily Healing Process Now

You can start now to formulate your own daily rituals which create new habits and new pathways in the brain and nervous system. Use the methods and tools described here to begin your healing journey. Get started. But first, breathe.

Your Next Steps

You can feel, dance, move, write, and journal yourself into joy, peace, hope, and gratitude, but you need to work with someone who can help you release the trapped energy inside your body, in a group or private setting.

Take the Next Step to Healing

We have talked about how to release trauma and discussed some ways you can help yourself start the healing process with breathing, movement, writing, and other exercises. If you would like to take this further and do deeper work, I want to share with you how to turn this immediately useful information into lasting healing and transformation.

There are tools, training, and support for you!

I want to encourage you to work with someone to help you get the healing results you need, so you can return to living a healthy, joyful life.

These are the steps you need to take to get the results that are possible for you, whether you do it with me or with another practitioner who has similar training and does similar work.

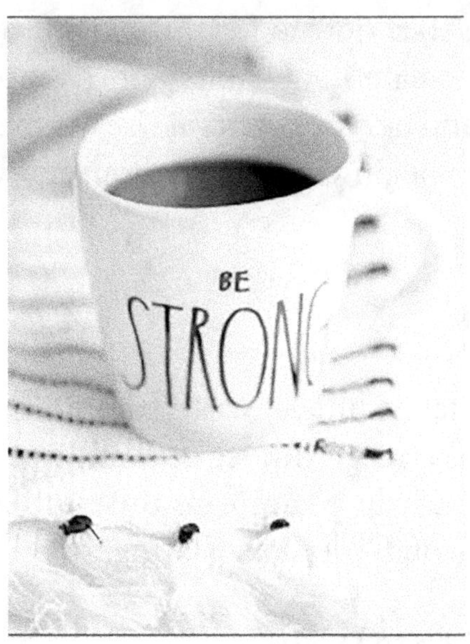

Know your strength. You are stronger than you realize.

Do Breathwork

Commit to yourself to a series of 10 breathwork sessions to start. Once you master the technique, do 15 to 20 minutes of 100 conscious, connected breaths each day. This maintenance can be your daily meditation or part of it.

Healing is a journey, not accomplished by just one breathwork session, especially if you have years of suffering from emotional pain, physical problems, long-standing life problems, or past, chronic, ongoing, or intensive trauma— but this is the quickest, most effective, and lasting way, at least for me and innumerous others around the world, and does not require years of expensive extensive psychoanalysis and therapy, diagnostic testing, and risky treatment that has serious side effects.

Rebirth Yourself

Rebirth Yourself

The benefits of optimal breathing are well documented. Let your Clarity Breathwork sessions give you the tools to:

1. Heal your emotional wounds and traumas in a way that lasts (to feel like yourself again—or even better!).
2. Break the cycle of chronic inner stress and adrenalized states, reduce inner stress, feel incredible relief, lighter and more comfortable in your body, and easily navigate stressful situations and difficult challenges with resilience.
3. Reap the rewards of anti-aging, cellular detoxification, a stronger immune system, decreased inflammation, reduced blood pressure, and better sleep and overall health.
4. Improve your focus and concentration.
5. Enhance exercise and sports performance.
6. Lead a richer, more fulfilled and purposeful life.
7. Feel increased aliveness, energy, and vitality, and have more ease and flow in your life.
8. Remove what feels like immovable blocks and transform negative or self-limiting beliefs, thought patterns, habits, and behaviors that stand in your way to living the life you want.

9. Have greater emotional intelligence, clarity, a deeper sense of knowing, and profound insights into your core life's issues, decisions, and unique gifts.
10. Cultivate acceptance, understanding, reconciliation, and even gratitude for past hurts—and see the gifts in your story.
11. Enhance forgiveness, compassion, and love for yourself and others.
12. Take responsibility for your life, your inner joy, and peace—no matter what challenges you face.
13. Connect to your spirituality, with the true magnificence of who you are, your bigger purpose and vision for your life; restore your self-worth and value in this world.
14. Connect to and feel the benefits of a community, develop deep, lasting, authentic friendships with others who are going through similar experiences of healing from pain, transformational growth, and reclamation of joy.

Say YES to yourself! *I'm ready to take down what's holding me back from living the happy, fulfilled, and abundant life that is my birthright.*

Begin reclaiming your inner calm and joyful, fulfilled, and abundant life right away!

Contact me or another similar Breathwork Practitioner for more information about scheduling your sessions.

I can't wait for you to feel huge healing and transformation in your life, the miracles I myself have experienced and witnessed. When I think about my decision point to commit to healing, personal growth, and transforming through breathwork and immersing myself in a series of sessions, I am brought to tears of gratitude.

In the modern world where it has never been acceptable to fully feel and express our full range of emotions, being REAL, transformational healing, and living in full joy are revolutionary acts. My mission is to empower you to heal from inner stress, pain, and trauma that has held you back in all aspects of your life, live in a relaxed state of joy, flow, resilience, and fulfillment, and healthy authentic emotional expression safe for all—in the world that urgently needs us to heal, bring ourselves and others higher, and show up fully with our gifts. Let's heal and learn to let ourselves shine together!

Top 5 Questions About Clarity Breathwork and Trauma Release

Five Top Questions About Clarity Breathwork and Trauma Release

I know you are feeling fear and hesitation because I and others have felt it too. I want you to know this work CHANGED AND SAVED my life, and I want this for you too. Let me answer the top five questions and concerns people present to me before jumping into Clarity Breathwork. Then, if you have further questions, you can always contact me or another similar breathworker directly.

1—I am afraid of my pain; to revisit the past and my trauma.

If you are reading this book, you are in some degree of pain and suffering. First of all, you are in good hands—I have either felt or seen it all as a human being, midwife, and Certified Clarity Breathwork Practitioner. I have healed myself and have helped others heal. No emotional pain is too big or dangerous.

I know what the darkest and lowest is all too well, ten on a scale of one to ten. I have been there and came out on the other side from this work only.

I tried it all as I told you. This work is completely safe without risks, other than healing, feeling so much better beyond your wildest imagination, back to yourself if you can remember what that was like, in delicious relief, joy and calm, creating a life you love. What could be better?

We live in a culture that is not comfortable with discomfort and pain, and encourages escape, denial, keeping it in, or numbing. Pain calls us to listen for the messages; to take important action. Your body does not lie. Pain is, indeed, inevitable, but suffering, how we react, and the stories we tell ourselves about the sensations we feel, is optional. In this world, there is sun and rain, light and dark, joy and pain. They are all needed, essential to living, and are all sacred/holy essential parts of our being. Feeling all feelings leads to living fully in our greatest potential.

When doing this work, the invitation is to allow, surrender, let go, relax into, love, and embrace all sensations and feelings, even if it seems at times—especially early on—not comfortable or downright intense and overwhelming. "Bring it on" is the ideal mindset, as there lies your freedom.

Stay present and open and curious, but the main thing is, dive right in, let it all be as it is, but most important: keep breathing … and relaxing into intensity.

Know you are safe and supported and loved by those who support and love you—including your spiritual guide(s). Your certified well-trained breathworker is there with you, holding space, guiding and supporting you, but we do not try to fix, change, or suppress you—as that interferes. You can draw on unseen or your own internal support. You are stronger than you think. You have the innate power to heal yourself, if given the opportunity and the tools. YOU are bigger than any pain, fear, or memory.

What events occurred in the past have already passed and are not happening now. What is happening are the results of your trapped pain and trauma. Your recurring self-limiting thought patterns are robbing you of your present. The healing and transformation is in the feeling, letting go, surrendering, and trusting the process, your body's infinite wisdom to process, reset, and release what is not serving you.

All is confidential—we breathworkers create boundaries—we all agree what goes on in the private or group sessions stays in the sessions.

As in the heat of birth (a normal and healthy huge transformation), during the most intense sensations of late labor and as the baby is crowning/emerging, many women tell me they can't, it is too much, they want a cesarean, they think something is really wrong, they panic, think they will explode, go crazy, even die, and they tend to fight it. It is when they are reassured all is well, reminded to tap into their strength they did not know they had, they pray to a higher power, stop resisting, let go, surrender to the brilliant process that is far wiser than any human, they go with it and ride the waves; then they give birth.

Every time. The same happens in breathwork sessions, healing, and rebirthing.

Resistance is common and means you are going in the right direction. If you start thinking, "This isn't working, I don't like it, it's too hard, I am not doing it right, it is easier to just stay where I am/what I'm used to"—even if your life is not working, you feel terrible suffering and dis-ease—welcome it, know those are all signs to keep on going, keep breathing. What you resist persists and only increases your suffering. No one said it would be easy, but it sure is worth it.

2—I don't have the time or money. I'm too busy, and I can't afford it.

I felt that way, too, before I took the initial leap and invested in my healing. It was about what was my priority. I made time and money for what I valued, and this was a necessity for me. What I am aware of from being in this field and working with so many suffering humans is the extent of pain you feel and its impact on your life, that two hours once a week or every other week times ten, and even with a daily ritual self-care practice—it is a blip in the grand scheme of things.

If I added up the years, the energy, everything I spent on all sorts of ineffective treatments, therapies, and remedies with all sorts of providers and therapists, plus the books, workshops, and retreats—it is overwhelmingly huge; how do you measure the cost, time, and energy of terrible suffering? The inner pain and torture? The not feeling fully alive and well? The life and relationship problems, self-sabotaging and limiting yourself, and getting in your own way?

Let me ask you: what is it costing you in time, money, energy, peace of mind, joy, fulfillment, relationships, work/career by not doing this? How much time, money, energy, vitality, and opportunity do you lose daily, weekly, monthly, and yearly by not healing and continuing to suffer from this pain and inner stress you have had for years?

Let me tell you—the way I feel now is priceless. I would have paid anything and spent whatever time/energy that was needed had I known about it sooner.

When I look back at my decision to make the investment for my own   Breathwork sessions and workshops, it was worth more than every dollar, every minute spent. I am just so grateful/thankful to my younger self that she had the courage to make that decision. Because of her, I am back to myself, healed fully, living in my inner calm and joy, so full and fulfilled that I am able to give back and help you and others birth and rebirth themselves and have that same experience. That is what I want for you.

3—What if I need personal help, how will I get that in an online or group session?

I thought that too, but some of my most powerful healing sessions were in a group. There is an option for private sessions—I did both and felt I needed both, but most do just fine in group sessions. And many benefit immensely by private sessions, in person or online. There are centers all over the world sometimes as common as yoga studios, where people go to breathe in a group regularly.

The benefits of a group are many—knowing you are not alone can help heal the wound of illusion of separation; hearing and witnessing others' experiences can help validate your own and you realize your pain/divinity in others/their pain and divinity in yours; the universality of pain and wounds comforts as you see that how you reacted to what you faced is normal and more common than you imagined; knowing we are all in this together is also comforting; if anyone needs help, they speak up and ask for it.

The breathworker is there with you throughout, and many have assistants in larger groups. We all hear and see each other, so the support and guidance given to one can apply to all. So let it in and see how it benefits you. If something releases from one of you, it heals and releases from all. Receiving support like honest, loving feedback and observations can accelerate your growth and transformation.

Connecting in a conscious, supportive, loving community to people like yourself, where vulnerability and authenticity are the norm, often begins in the relationship with a professional practitioner. It can lead to profound healing. Some of my greatest friendships that last to this day are from those I met and connected with in my group workshops. We need real community in this age of high-tech isolation.

There is plenty of opportunity to maintain this connection on the private Facebook groups and beyond, but I encourage more nourishing connections in person as opposed to social media. You get out of it what you put into it.

I also do have a spiritual perspective and trust that we are all held and supported. We call on the support of our guides, mentors, our biggest support staff, alive or not, angels, the divine. I trust we are held by the beloved and supported. That nothing will come up that you or an experienced breathworker cannot handle. And again, you can opt for private one-on-one sessions. While in-person is preferable to online, as we benefit so much from actual connection and human comforting touch, there is still connection and breath-workers can offer support and healing touch with their words. The online option is great for those who can not travel and do not have access to a local practitioner. The session can be just as powerful, as the breath is really the main event.

4—What if I don't trust myself to do the work?

If you don't trust yourself to get on a two-hour group session, private in-person or online session, one time a week or every other week for ten weeks, and make some transformative lifestyle changes—then this may not be for you or you may not be ready yet to heal and transform your life. But, if you are ready to have healing breakthroughs, and this is calling you, plow through your resistance. Resistance, as I said, is a great sign to welcome. And you will be welcome where you are.

5—Will this really work for me?

A common question I get and I had myself was "What if it doesn't work for me? I've tried so many things and nothing has helped. Nothing works for me, why would this?" Another is "I do breathwork exercises in yoga" or "I have done rebirthing or holotropic breathwork before and didn't like it."

"Nothing will work for me" is a limiting, untrue thought. The opposite is usually more true—"What if it does work for me?" Try that on and imagine how it feels. Imagine what it feels like to heal, to not have your suffering, to feel joy and relief and calm. To love your life.

There are no guarantees to anything, but again, I also tried just about everything and nothing worked before for me either, but this worked for me completely and has lasted to this day, as I told you. It saved my life and those of so many others I have witnessed. This is powerful work like no other I had experienced.

It is not at all yoga pranayama breathing exercises, which are wonderful and have their place. This is a specific form of breathwork to heal the trapped energy of inner stress, dysfunctional repetitive thinking, inner stress, pain, and trauma.

I do not know what type of breathwork you did, what training your practitioner had, or what support was given. This is a unique revolutionary approach, an art, and a science, that works for those who are ready and eager to do it, to play full-out. The only thing in your way is yourself. We often get in our own way. It is time for healing, freedom, and joy beyond your expectations and what you think is possible! I invite you to step up! I know you can do this!

A Critical Part of Lifestyle Medicine

Address any undetected body dysfunction that can cause many symptoms of mental illness and other common ailments to ensure you are physiologically in balance and healthy. This could be from medication and drug side effects and toxic exposures in food, water, body care products, household products, and your environment; chronic inflammation, blood sugar, hormone, and gut flora imbalance, nutritional deficiencies; isolation or insufficient exercise, sleep, nature, or sun exposure.

Taking excellent care of your body is part of healing and ensures your body is optimally functioning while you are on your trauma- and life-healing path. Your body is brilliantly resilient, perfectly designed to repair itself and feel great when given the opportunity. According to cutting-edge evidence-based lifestyle medicine, putting unhealthy or toxic products into your body, chronic stress exposure, and lack of adequate nutrition, activity, time in nature, sun, or sleep takes a huge toll on health and wellbeing. The wonderful news is that you can absolutely do it, and the effects are as profound in the body as breath is in your being. And it is all interconnected.

Take it on as an opportunity to get curious and wonder about the miraculous being that you are, what your wise body is communicating. Listen carefully and make needed changes. It could be as simple as a few blood tests with an integrative practitioner to check thyroid function and antibodies, cortisol, blood sugar screen, vitamin B12 and D levels, and adding needed supplements to support body function, immunity, and detoxification, and to reduce excess inflammation or balance hormones. It could be as simple as detoxing your diet and environment, drinking ample clean water, reducing stress, mastering your relaxation response, getting better sleep, regular exercise, increased time outside in nature and sunshine, and more nurturing, meaningful connections with others. Many do and feel best on an organic Paleo diet, off gluten, dairy, cane sugar, high fructose corn syrup and artificial sweeteners, corn, soy, refined vegetable oils and processed, chemically-laden products, and genetically modified organisms (GMOs)–eating plenty of non-inflammatory, nutrient-dense whole-plant foods, animal protein, and healthy fats. This is more in line with how our healthier ancestors ate for thousands of years– what they hunted and gathered.

For more details on natural lifestyle suggestions and remedies for optimal health and wellbeing, refer to my Natural Birth Secrets book, as there I cover this in detail. Even if you are not pregnant, much of it still applies and is relevant to all.

For those who want to dive into the science and research, as well as follow a structured program that has effectively helped thousands, read integrative psychiatrist Kelly Brogan's two books listed in the references–*A Mind of Your Own and Own Your Self;* for even more support, take her online Vital Mind Reset course.

Moving out of victimhood and taking radical responsibility for your health and wellbeing are the first steps to resolving your problems and reclaiming your whole-body health. What is amazing is that it's totally within your control! Now that's super empowering and beyond hopeful.

About the Author

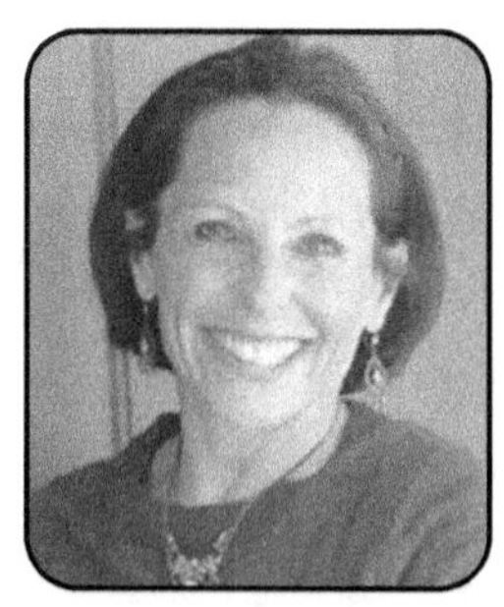

Anne Margolis
CNM, LM, MSN,
BSN, RNC

Anne Margolis is a Licensed Certified Nurse Midwife, Licensed Femme! Teacher, Certified Clarity Breathwork Practitioner, and Yoga Teacher and practitioner. Anne is a third-generation guide to mamas birthing babies in her family. Anne has helped thousands of families in her 24-plus-year midwifery practice and has personally ushered the births of over 1,000 healthy babies into the world. She has also guided countless human beings to heal from emotional pain, inner stress, and trauma, and to tap into their strength and power, live fully and vibrantly, and reclaim their radiance, joyfulness, calm, and overall sense of wellbeing.

Through her online childbirth course "Love Your Birth," her online and in-person midwifery for pregnancy and postpartum support consultations, her birth professional mentoring, her holistic gynecology, Clarity Breathwork offerings, and Femme! experience offerings, Anne infuses wisdom, compassion, inspiration, and joy into the entire process of women's healthcare—from teen-aged years to menopause. Anne also facilitates incredible healing and wellness for both men and women of all ages.

Anne is a two-time number one national and international best-selling author of this book and also Natural Birth Secrets. Anne's work, insights, and advice have been featured on TV shows and movies, including four episodes of A Baby Story on TLC Discovery Channel, the award-winning feature documentary *Orgasmic Birth*, and *The Human Longevity Project.*

Anne has also been a featured speaker and expert panelist at distinguished events for Weil-Cornell School of Medicine, the University of Pennsylvania School of Nursing, RCC State University of New York School of Nursing, Birthnet Association of Childbirth Professionals, and Hudson Valley Birth Network, to name a few.

Anne's Clarity Breathwork and Femme! healing movement workshops have been hosted at several yoga studios and wellness centers, including the conscious, high vibration, and transformational community at The Assemblage in New York City. Anne is a proud founding member of The Health and Wellness Business Association, which was created to promote initiatives that support better collaboration, interaction, and ethical business practices within the health and wellness business community.

Anne has midwifed mamas and babies for over two decades and guides individuals to birth themselves as healthy and whole human beings capable of immense joy and inner peace. Her clients describe her as "passionate," "sensitive," "big-hearted," and a "playful ball of light." When she's not helping mamas around the world, you can find her doing yoga (anywhere and everywhere), dancing, taking or facilitating powerful growth and healing workshops, traveling, enjoying family time, and watching historical dramas and comedies.

Learn more now and get started on your healing journey today.
http://homesweethomebirth.com/clarity-breathwork-new-york

References

Kelly Brogan, MD. *A Mind of Your Own, The Truth About Depression and How Women Can Heal Their Bodies and Reclaim Their Lives.* Thorsons, an imprint of HarperCollins Publishers, 2016.

Kelly Brogan, MD. *Own Your Self: The Surprising Path Beyond Depression, Anxiety, and Fatigue to Reclaiming Your Authenticity, Vitality, and Freedom.* Hay House Inc., 2019.

Kelly Brogan, MD. *https://kellybroganmd.com/in-honor-of-fear-and-pain/*

Dan Brule. *Breath Mastery Fundamentals Workbook,* 2019.

Dan Brule. *Just Breathe: Mastering Breathwork.* Enliven/Atria, an imprint of Simon & Schuster, 2017.

Lauren Chelec Cafritz. *Breath Love.* Warren Publishing, 2019.

Dana Delong, Peter Delongm, and Ashanna Solaris. *Clarity Breathwork Training Manuals Levels 1–4.* ClarityBreathwork. com, 2018.

Judith Kravitz. *Breathe Deep Laugh Loudly: The Joy of Transformational Breathing.* Free Birth Press, 2007.

Judith Kravitz. *Transformational Breath Personal Seminar–Levels 1, 2 & 3.* 2014.

Peter Levine. *In an Unspoken Voice: How the Body Releases Trauma and Restores Goodness.* North Atlantic Books, 2010.

Ela Manga, MD. *Breathe: Strategizing Energy in the Age of Burnout.* MFBooks, Joburg, 2018.

Christiane Northrup, MD.   *https://www.drnorthrup.com/premenstrual-syndrome/*

Regina Thomashauer. *Mama Gena's School of Womanly Arts.* Simon & Schuster, 2002.

Regina Thomashauer. *Pussy, A Reclamation.* Hay House Inc., 2016.

Andrew Weil, MD. *Breathing: The Master Key to Self Healing.*

Journal Notes

Anne Margolis | 176